Authorization to Copy

Please feel free to copy any sections of
the book to give to patients or families
for informational purposes.

Author

Schizophrenia

A Guide for Patients, their Families, and Clinicians

Tirath S Gill MD

Contributions by

Prof. Paramjeet Singh MD

Father John Theophane OCD

"I think playing somebody who's schizophrenic is such a lesson as an actor. It gets you totally out of your comfort zone because you can't rely on your technique, your external stuff. You've really gotta look inward, in a way."

Matt Dillon

DISCLAIMER

No book can replace the services of a qualified mental health professional. Please use this book to help you communicate more effectively with your doctor so that you can obtain the best possible care. This book is not a guide for self-medication. The treatment of schizophrenia and schizoaffective disorder is a complex enterprise that requires collaboration between different professionals. The author and publisher disclaim responsibility for any misapplication of the information contained in this book.

Dedication

Dr. A Prettipaul PsyD

ACKNOWLEDGEMENTS

Many colleagues have contributed to our knowledge and insights about schizophrenia and schizoaffective disorder.

Much of the advice that we received is only acquired through hard-earned clinical experience over many years. Many have shared their wisdom.

In particular, I would like to acknowledge Dr. Hani Khouzam, Dr. Al Howsepian, Barbara Noyce RN, Dr. Beverely Sutton, Dr. Sarabjeet Aujla (Late), Dr. Robert Withrow, Dr. Michael Golding, Dr. Simarjit Gill, Dr. Ed Kaftarian, Dr. Roger Lyons, Dr. Godwin Ugwueze Dr. Kulwant Singh, Dr. Melinda Diciro, and Dr Aakash Ahuja. Other notable clinicians include Dr. Suresh Balani, Dr. Ravi Chand, Dr. Daulat Singh, Dr. Jaskaran Sandhu and Dr. Amar Chawla. Last but not least, Father John Theophane also shared his insights about working through compassion with the mentally ill in chronic care institutions. Professor Paramjeet Singh has offered his unique perspectives on difficult clinical situations. There may be controversial views in this book. These are mine and not attributable to any of the above clinicians.

Dr. Prettipaul has shared his struggles to help a loved one afflicted with this illness. I have been struck by his compassion and advocacy for the mentally ill. I told him I would write something and dedicate it to him, and so it is.

Many other wonderful people, too numerous to mention, also contributed to a better understanding of schizophrenia and closely related clinical conditions. I thank them all.

TSG

PREFACE

This book offers an overview of the illness of schizophrenia. Its objective is to offer hope if you or your loved one suffers from schizophrenia. It contains information that can provide guidance in obtaining relief for the symptoms that cause distress.

The truth is that schizophrenia is very treatable, and much can be done to reduce the symptoms and suffering of the individual.

At the end of the book, I have included a glossary of common psychiatric terms. I encourage you to look at it even before you read the rest of the book and whenever you have to again. It will be useful for understanding the book more fully if you are unfamiliar with the traditional psychiatric concepts. In the beginning, I have included some history that is relevant to the current understanding of schizophrenia.

I have tried to keep the language conversational and avoided jargon whenever possible. The language may still seem convoluted at times; I apologize for this in advance.

Some of the sections are very basic, and some sections may be a bit too detailed for the lay reader. Most of the concepts, however, are not beyond the ken and understanding of the dedicated reader.

Incidently, many of the concepts discussed here also apply to the closely related illness of schizoaffective disorder. The main difference is the need often for an additional mood stabilizer such as lithium or valproic acid (Depakote) when treating schizoaffective disorder.

Each chapter and each question-answer segment are self-contained, so feel free to stop anywhere and skip to what interests you. You don't have to read the book from beginning to end to derive some benefit from your reading. Sometimes the pronoun he or him may be used for convenience. Most of the advice in the book applies to both men and women.

I hope the information in this book will be helpful to you as I meant it to be. Some sections may be repetitious. There is a method to it.

Please feel free to leave a comment in the review section of the book. Your opinion is valuable.

TSG

CONTENTS

CHAPTER 1

A BRIEF HISTORY OF PSYCHOSIS AND SCHIZOPHRENIA

Schizophrenia is the illness that fits most people's idea of mental illness. It is an illness that has been recognized since ancient times and antiquity. The written record goes back to the ancient Egyptian period of the upper and lower Nile civilizations.

Psychosis is described in ancient Egyptian texts such as the Ebers papyrus dating back to 1500 BC. In this document titled "The Book of Hearts," mental illness is described with symptoms similar to schizophrenia. It was titled the "The Book of Hearts" because human thoughts were thought to reside in the heart and not in the head.

The next great throng of humanity to awaken out of the darkness was the Greek civilization. It gave us the noble physician Hippocrates and sublime philosophers such as Plato, Aristotle and others. Hippocrates was a highly ethical and humble physician and is revered as the father of modern medicine. He lived between 460 and 377 BC or about 2400 years ago. He advocated for the compassionate treatment of the mentally ill.

The philosopher Plato recognized that the brain was the source of our emotions. This is exemplified in a quote attributed to him: "Only from the brains springs our pleasures, our feelings of happiness, laughter and jokes, our pain, our sorrows, and tears.... This same organ makes us mad or confused, inspires us with fear."

Aristotle, the teacher of Alexander the Great, followed Plato, and also advocated an illness view of mental illness.

Christianity came on the scene a little over 2000 years ago. It ascribed evil spirits to be the cause of mental illness. In the New Testament, a man is described who meets some criteria for mental illness. He is reported to live at the edge of the town in isolation and engage in odd behaviors such as harming himself.

Because of the strange symptoms that mental illness can produce, it arouses anxiety and fear in some people. Due to such mindsets, many societies separated and ostracized individuals with mental illness.

The lack of support and abandonment by the larger group usually meant certain death due to the elements or by wildlife.

There were, however, remarkable exceptions to such callousness. In some societies, individuals with unusual symptoms were revered and cared for. They were regarded as special and referred to as being "afflicted by the divine." Many were treated with compassion in areas of the Middle East, India, Asia, and Africa.

The person suffering from unusual perceptions and behaviors was at times even elevated to the rank of a monk, shaman, or priest.

This continues even today in many cultures.

In the first and second centuries, the Roman physician Asclepiades and philosopher Cicero (106-43 BC) were influential. Up until then, the four humor theory of illness was prevalent. They asserted that mental illness stemmed not from the imbalance of the humors but from emotions such as rage, grief, and fear.

As happens in history, progress takes two steps forward and one step back. A later Roman physician, Celsus, became influential thereafter and began to preach a more backward and superstitious notion that mental illness was a punishment from God.

The Roman Empire was in full sway at that time. When Emperor Constantine adopted Christianity, it became the state religion. The empire spread the views of Celsus and Christianity about the demonic origins of mental illness. Prayers, purgatives, and bloodletting were the main tools of treatment.

Some hapless individuals in the throes of their illness were deemed demons, witches, warlocks, and heretics. The usual punishment for this was death by burning at the stake or by other means. This went on till as late as the Salem witch trials in 1692-1693.

In the middle ages, around 1500 AD, an age of reform began. Brave priests, monks, and other theologians questioned the old dogma and advocated a more compassionate view towards those with mental illness. Many monasteries were offered for the housing and treatment of the mentally ill.

Other institutions like the Bethlehem hospital began to house individuals who suffered from serious illnesses such as schizophrenia and schizoaffective disorder. (See Footnote)

In the 17th century, good sense prevailed through the idea that mental illness was related to biology, stressful emotions, and trauma. John Locke, Denis Diderot and the famous physician Phillippe Pinel (1745-1826) were the foremost amongst these pioneers that forged a way out of the darkness.

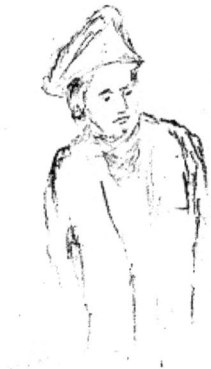

Dr. Philippe Pinel instructs staff to strike down the chains of the mentally ill

Dr. Phillippe Pinel is respectfully remembered as the one who advocated openly for the humane treatment of the mentally ill. He is famous for having struck down the chains of chronically ill patients at the Salpêtrière Hospital in Paris. He eloquently spoke about the treatment of the mentally ill with respect and kindness. He was also one of the first to advance the idea that there should be some level of confidentiality in treatment by a doctor. In addition, he advocated for the creation of calm environments in which to treat patients. He also set up routine, structured programs and activities to achieve a therapeutic benefit. His model of treatment became the basis of the moral treatment of mental illness.

Other notable reformers of this age who advocated for the moral treatment of the mentally ill were William Tuke in England and Benjamin Rush, the father of American psychiatry in the United States.

Incidentally, Benjamin Rush was also one the founding fathers of the United States. He was one of the original signers of the Declaration of Independence.

William Tuke founded the York Institute based on the above model of moral treatment. It became the template for other asylums built in England and the United States in the 19th century.

THE ADVENT AND DECLINE OF LARGE STATE HOSPITALS

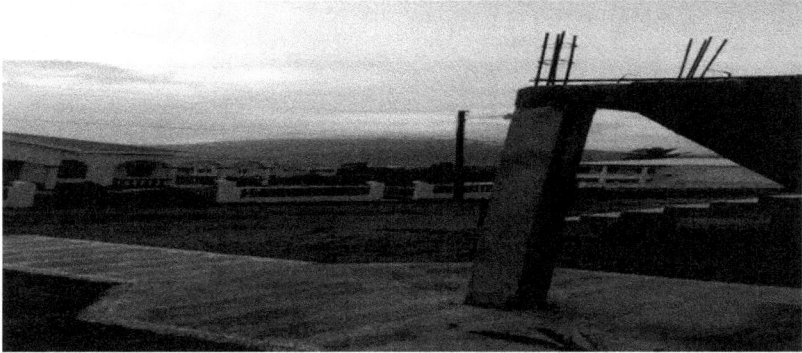

Large psychiatric hospitals were first built in Pennsylvania by the Christian Quaker community to house individuals with chronic mental illness. The asylums were built on the model of moral treatment advocated by Phillippe Pinel and William Tuke.

The federal and state governments then picked up the interest in housing the mentally ill. They launched one of the biggest building projects of the 19th century.

The building of large state hospitals in the 19th century has been compared in its grand scope to the building of the interstate highway system under President Eisenhower in the 1950s. It was built at considerable public expense to house the chronically mentally ill in supportive settings.

Many states had realized that the mentally ill were wandering in the countryside without proper shelter or care.

In some ways, the completion of this project represented the best ideals of a young democracy with its compassion for the less fortunate.

Elaborate programs were set up for the patients at the state hospitals to help them earn self-respect. Trade skills and education were provided to those who were trainable. Every attempt was made to normalize life for individuals housed at these institutions.

There were even annual balls and banquets that were graced by high society gentlemen and ladies. The individual patients were also provided work in small farms run by the hospitals. This was based on the ideas of Pinel of providing structure and meaningful work.

In some cities, the state hospital was spread out over many acres and housing was even provided free for the many staff that worked there. The hospitals also provided useful educational opportunities for the training of nurses, medical professionals, and mental health professionals. Many state hospitals were large enough to have their own zip codes.

In 1952, a medication going by the brand name of Thorazine was introduced. The generic name of this revolutionary medication was chlorpromazine, and it provided, for the first time, a means of reliably treating symptoms of schizophrenia.

The results were truly remarkable, and many hospital wards full of disturbed, agitated patients started to become calmer. This calming was achieved through a real reduction in psychotic symptoms and not merely through the sedation that it also provided.

In the subsequent years, other antipsychotics were introduced. Many social activists advocated for the release of individuals from the state hospitals.

The result was that thousands of former state hospital patients were gradually released to return to the communities where they had originally come from. Local community mental health centers were set up to continue the psychiatric care of these and other individuals in the community.

Many patients were able to integrate back into the community. This was often dependent on the level of support they had in the community.

Those who had poor support drifted towards homelessness. Many were convicted of minor or major crimes in their psychiatrically unstable state and imprisoned in jails and prisons.

This quagmire persists and remains our current state of affairs. Many individuals who would have earlier been in a state hospital are now in prisons. The prisons have become the defacto state hospitals of yesteryear.

The prison population has, in fact, been exploding. This is due to harsher laws, mandatory sentences and also due to the collapse of social support structures in the community for those with serious mental illness.

The future will hopefully bring greater funding for community treatment centers. Also, it is possible that some former state hospitals will be reopened again and run in a humanitarian manner.

Footnote: The word "bedlam" became an adjective to imply a chaotic, loud and disorganized state of affairs representative of the scene at Bethlehem hospital where many individuals with psychosis were housed without the benefit of effective treatments.

Many people were amused by the seemingly chaotic goings-on at Bethlehem hospital and tickets were even sold to the public to view the din and noise of the institution. The concept of privacy was still not well defined, and the rights of the mentally ill had still not been fully defined.

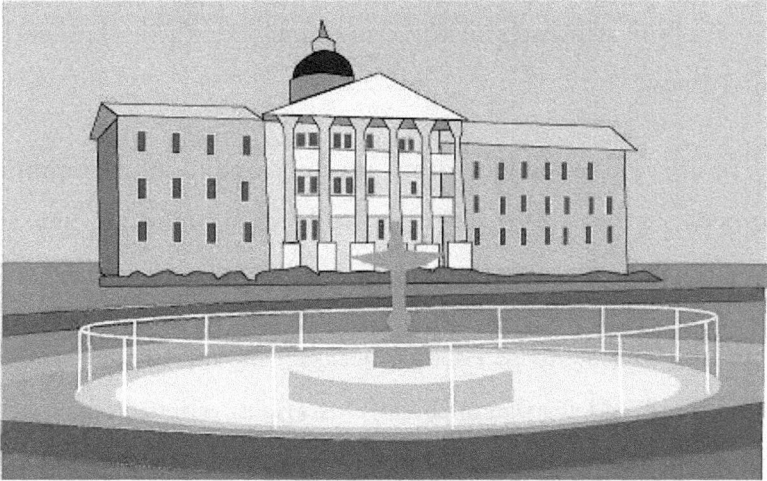

A drawing of Austin State Hospital Administration Building where I trained. The rest of the hospital is spread out over many acres in the heart of Austin, Texas.

CHAPTER 2

UNDERSTANDING SCHIZOPHRENIA

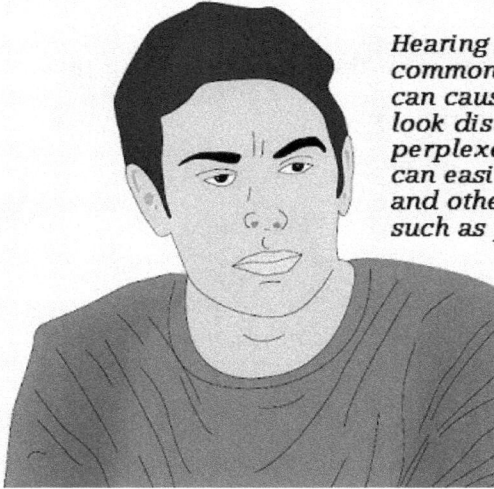

Hearing of Voices is a common symptom. It can cause a person to look distracted and perplexed. Medications can easily control this and other symptoms such as fearful feelings.

Most Symptoms can be reduced with meds in one to two weeks

Schizophrenia is a disabling brain disorder that, by definition, lasts for a period of six months or longer. The illness affects many functions of the brain including the expression of emotions and the processing of thoughts. If not treated, the illness can make it difficult for the person to carry on relationships and sustain productivity at work. Schizophrenia is marked by a loss of touch with reality and is accompanied by various symptoms such as the hearing of voices (hallucinations) and delusions (false fixed beliefs).

SCHIZOPHRENIA CRITERIA FROM DSM 5

Following are the main criteria for the diagnosis of schizophrenia from the DSM5:

Criteria A:

Two or more symptoms from the following list are present for at least one month (less if treated):

Delusions

Hallucinations

Disorganized behaviors

Disorganized speech

Negative symptoms (flattening of emotional expression - flat affect, alogia - decreased speech, avolition - decreased drive to do anything)

Criteria B:

Social and Occupational Dysfunction is present. This can be evidenced by a decreased ability for self-care, or a decreased ability to get along with others. There may also be a decreased ability to work or maintain their prior level of productivity. This global decline is a decrease from the previous level of functioning.

Criteria for Duration: The symptom duration should be at least six months.

Criteria of Exclusion: The symptoms are not related to Substance Abuse, Schizoaffective Disorder, Medical Disorder or Mood Disorder with psychotic features.

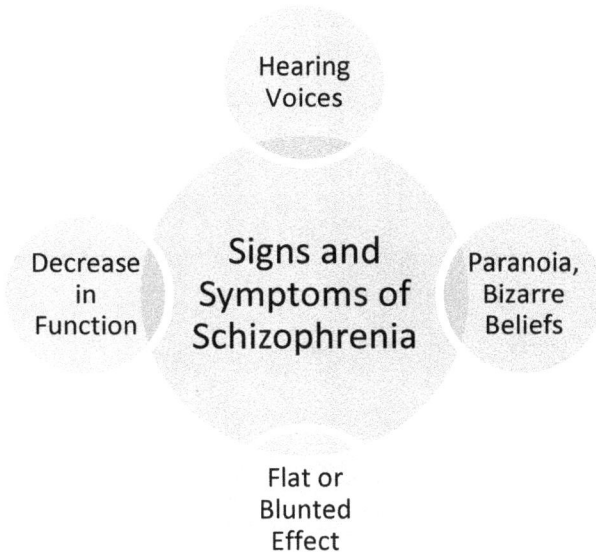

Hearing
Voices

Decrease
in
Function

Signs and
Symptoms of
Schizophrenia

Paranoia,
Bizarre
Beliefs

Flat or
Blunted
Effect

AT WHAT AGE DO THE SYMPTOMS OF SCHIZOPHRENIA START TO MANIFEST THEMSELVES?

The symptoms of schizophrenia usually start in the early twenties. The onset can be gradual and over many months, or it may come on rapidly in a matter of days and weeks.

Prevalence: The prevalence of schizophrenia is about 1%.

Prevalence of all psychotic illness is about 3 percent

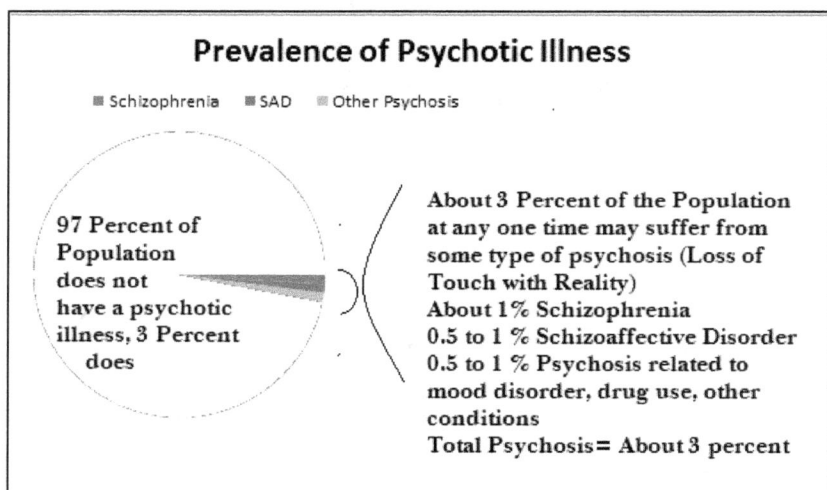

Prevalence of Psychotic Illness

■ Schizophrenia   ■ SAD   ■ Other Psychosis

97 Percent of Population does not have a psychotic illness, 3 Percent does

About 3 Percent of the Population at any one time may suffer from some type of psychosis (Loss of Touch with Reality)
About 1% Schizophrenia
0.5 to 1 % Schizoaffective Disorder
0.5 to 1 % Psychosis related to mood disorder, drug use, other conditions
Total Psychosis= About 3 percent

RATIO OF PREVALENCE BETWEEN MEN AND WOMEN

The illness seems to affect men and women with equal frequency. The men come to attention sooner as they are more likely to be affected by their dysfunction at their job or school. The onset of illness in women was traditionally noted to have a later onset.

In the past, when these statistics were compiled, this may have had to do with the fact that many women did not go to college or join the workforce where dysfunction is more readily apparent. By their performance at home being under less scrutiny as compared to work or school, the incidence of dysfunction usually went undetected and unreported until it became severe in the later stages.

Another reason for the low reporting rates in women was the issue of stigma. It was considered a greater stigma for a woman to be deemed mentally ill, and this may have led families to underreport any mental illness in the women of the family.

In the current day and age, where opportunities for women have increased, there is an increasing recognition of mental illness in women at earlier ages. The age of onset of schizophrenia and the incidence of schizophrenia in men and women has been found to be similar and equal.

The onset of symptoms can be early as age 16, and most individuals with schizophrenia have symptoms by age 30. Cases earlier than age 16 are infrequent and also rare are new cases of schizophrenia after age 40.

If late or early onset symptoms of psychotic or mood symptoms are noted, a full medical workup should be done including an MRI or a CAT scan of the brain to rule out all medical causes.

PSYCHOSIS IN WOMEN

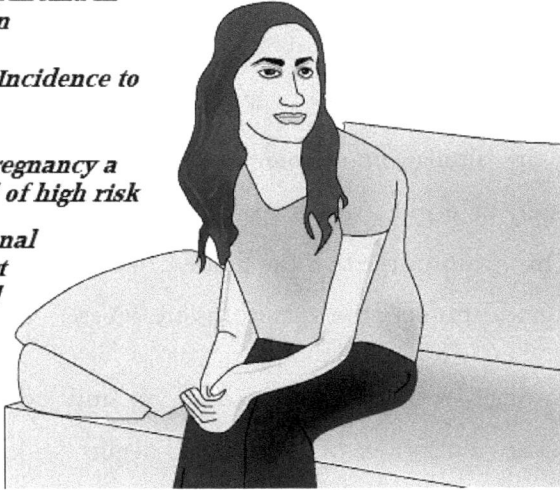

Schizophrenia in Women

Equal Incidence to Men

Post Pregnancy a period of high risk

Emotional Support Needed

ARE THERE DIFFERENCES IN THE PRESENTATION AND TREATMENT OF SCHIZOPHRENIA IN WOMEN?

The incidence and prevalence of schizophrenia and schizoaffective disorder are similar in women and men. The presentation in a woman may be noticed at a later age if choice or culture home bind them. The symptoms may be hidden, and dysfunction may not become evident unless the symptoms are severe.

The treatment response to medications and other measures is similar. The resolution of symptoms begins within a week and continues for the next few weeks after treatment is begun.

Some of the side effects related to medications are different in women patients. For example, there may be a change in the regularity of menstrual cycles.

Another side effect more likely in women is galactorrhoea. This is the production and leaking of breast milk. Galactorrhoea is caused by an elevation of the hormone prolactin. The elevation of prolactin is caused by a blockade of dopamine receptors in a small section of the brain called the hypothalamus. In men, elevation of prolactin may cause an increase in breast size; a condition called gynecomastia.

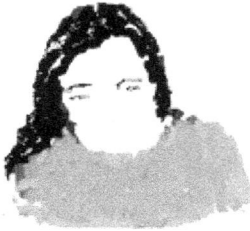

SCHIZOPHRENIA IN WOMEN

1. May be noticed at a later age.
2. May have menstrual irregularities with antipsychotic medications.
3. May need special adjustments of medications during pregnancy.
4. Breast feeding may be contraindicated if on antipsychotic medications.
5. Post partum period may be a period of high risk for relapse. Closer monitoring is helpful during this period

All antipsychotics have a risk for elevating prolactin. The risk may be less with antipsychotics such as quetiapine, aripiprazole, ziprasidone, lurasidone, and asenapine. Unfortunately, these antipsychotics don't always work for everyone, and some clinicians feel they are less effective as antipsychotics.

Olanzapine and clozapine are effective antipsychotics and may have less of a risk for increasing prolactin. They, however, carry more of a risk for causing metabolic syndrome (weight gain, elevation of cholesterol and elevation of blood sugars).

Clozapine is never used as first line antipsychotic and is held in reserve for refractory cases. This is due to the risk of bone marrow suppression that can occur in 1% of individuals that receive it.

Risperidone is an effective antipsychotic but has a tendency to cause significant elevations of prolactin in some individuals.

There is no perfect antipsychotic, and the decision has to be made by the patient and doctor in consultation with each other by weighing the potential benefits and risks of the medications.

When treating women, the doctor has to consider the risk of her getting pregnant, and the risk to her unborn child, carefully if she is on medication. For this reason, he may recommend birth control techniques to avoid unintended pregnancy. A planned pregnancy is safer for the mother and the child.

If the woman becomes pregnant, the doctor may reduce the dose of the medications in the first three months of her pregnancy. This is also called the first trimester, and it is during this period that the major organ systems in the baby are formed.

The reduction in medication dosage will reduce the risk of birth defects. Most medications tend to be safe, but caution is recommended with lithium, Depakote, and certain SSRI antidepressants such as paroxetine (Paxil).

The technical name for birth defects due to drugs or other environmental causes is teratogenesis.

Around the time of childbirth, when the mother delivers her baby, there are rapid shifts in body fluids and hormones. These can affect her mental health and doses of the medications will need to be carefully adjusted. If the medication doses were lowered during her pregnancy, they might need to be increased back to the previous stabilization doses.

In general, breastfeeding is contraindicated if the woman is on antipsychotic medications or mood stabilizers. The medications pass through the breast milk and can cause side effects in the infant.

The doctor will take a careful history of the symptoms, a history of any medical problems and also try to obtain a history of mental illness in other family members and their current social support structures. He or she will probably order some routine laboratory tests to rule out any major medical problems. This is similar to what would be done in the case of a male patient with schizophrenia.

IF SCHIZOPHRENIA IS PRESENT IN ONE TO TWO OUT OF EVERY 100 PEOPLE, WHY DON'T I SEE THEM WHEN I'M OUT IN THE COMMUNITY?

To some extent, the adage that the eye does not see what one does not know applies here. The other reasons why schizophrenia and schizoaffective disorder are not so frequently noticed in public is that most individuals with schizophrenia prefer to be alone and may not go to public settings.

Also, medications are quite effective in controlling the most prominent symptoms. This is a positive fact and a reason for hope as it shows that many individuals with this illness can function in society just like anyone else without calling attention to themselves. They are in every way as normal as anyone else and, in fact, may be more conscientious and more empathic than other individuals who have never suffered from illness.

A more somber reason individuals are not noticed is that some of them are locked up in prisons or jails if their illness gets bad and difficult to control. This usually is linked to some minor or major violation of the law. Some other individuals with more serious symptoms but noncriminal behaviors may reside in supportive settings such as group homes, state hospitals, and other inpatient settings.

Lastly, it must be understood that, although the incidence of schizophrenia is one percent, about 42% of the individuals may recover from the initial episode and never have a relapse again with treatment.

THE RANGE OF PSYCHOTIC SYMPTOMS

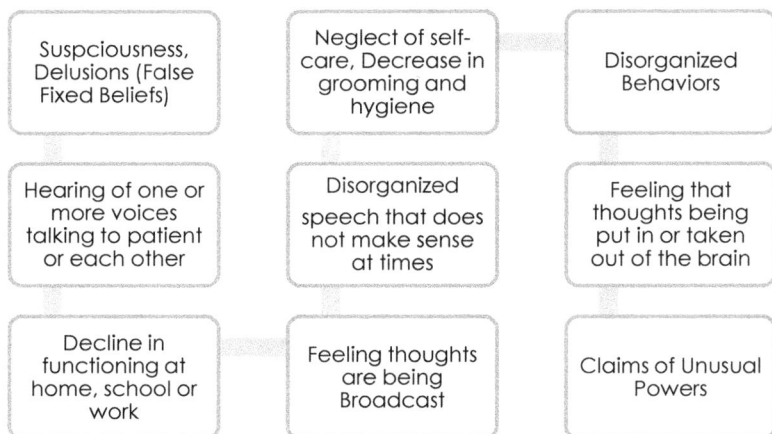

Suspciousness, Delusions (False Fixed Beliefs)	Neglect of self-care, Decrease in grooming and hygiene	Disorganized Behaviors
Hearing of one or more voices talking to patient or each other	Disorganized speech that does not make sense at times	Feeling that thoughts being put in or taken out of the brain
Decline in functioning at home, school or work	Feeling thoughts are being Broadcast	Claims of Unusual Powers

There are several different kind of psychotic symptoms, as illustrated in the above diagram, that can tie into one another.

Delusions are fixed false beliefs that are unshakable and impervious to logic. Delusions can develop around anything and can be varied. They may be bizarre and appear very strange to others but are very real to the person.

The delusions may be centered around the body (soma), and these are called somatic delusions. They may have an unusual somatic theme such as a controlling device being implanted into their body without their knowledge. This device is felt to generate voices to explain the auditory hallucinations that are generated by an excess of dopamine and other neurochemicals in the brain.

Sometimes the delusions are related to a sense of persecution by others. These beliefs are held with great tenacity and vigor. The person is not convinced by any amount of evidence that they may be wrong.

When treatment is begun, the delusions gradually wane in intensity and then gradually fade away with time. They tend to return when treatment is interrupted.

During a psychotic state, other psychotic symptoms may include hallucinations that seem very real. They may hear a voice when there is no one in the vicinity talking to them or anyone else. This is called an auditory hallucination (AH). The voice or voices generated by these hallucinations sound just like a voice from a real person and appear very real. It seems as if a real person is talking to them from behind a curtain or from somewhere unseen. The individual may look all around them to determine the source of the voice. When such a source is not found, the person may become deeply puzzled and perplexed. They may become agitated or may choose to ignore it and carry on.

In schizophrenia, other psychotic symptoms may include unintelligible speech, disorganized behaviors, odd posturing, and general neglect of self-care that is not related to depression.

It is not difficult to see how symptoms of schizophrenia can be very confusing and baffling for a person who is experiencing them and also for family and friends who have to watch their loved one decline in function. The decline in function is very real. It was the decline in functioning that led one of the pioneers of psychiatry, Emil Kraepelin, to label the illness to be a type of early dementia or dementia praecox.

The experience of developing psychosis can be frightening. In the words of one patient, it feels as if she is living in "a walking and waking nightmare."

HOW DOES THE ILLNESS OF SCHIZOPHRENIA NORMALLY BEGIN?

Many individuals that have schizophrenia describe feeling normal till one day when the first symptom makes its appearance as an odd experience. For example, they may be walking or doing something else when they hear something or someone speak to them. They may be startled and try to look around to figure out where the voice came from. Sometimes the individual may have become gradually withdrawn from others before the hallucinations make their appearance.

They may find it quite annoying and perplexing and wonder if someone is playing a prank on them. They may try to distract themselves by doing something else. The voice or voices may persist or sometimes may go away only to recur again at another unexpected moment.

The person may confide their unusual experience to someone such as a family members or friends who may be equally perplexed.

The family member or friend may ask them to speak to a doctor. They may have heard of some conditions such as tinnitus that can produce a tone or ringing in the ear. This condition of tinnitus is different, however, from the voices heard in schizophrenia and schizoaffective disorder. Some family members may be superstitious and think it to be a state of possession. They may try to consult a faith healer or shaman about the problem.

Many educated clergy and priests are informed about the role of treatable mental illness in causing bizarre symptoms and will refer the individual to a doctor for treatment.

The doctor, when told about these symptoms, will listen in a compassionate manner and recognize that these are symptoms of a treatable psychotic illness. He or she may start some antipsychotic medications and will most likely run some laboratory tests to rule out medical issues. The doctor may also run a urine drug screen to rule out the role of drugs in causing these frightening symptoms.

All doctors are trained to some degree in psychiatric diagnosis and treatment. Medical schools have made it an issue of greater focus in the training of doctors. This is because the bulk of psychiatric treatment across the world is provided by general practitioners and not by psychiatrists.

So your family doctor is probably familiar with the salient features of schizophrenia and bipolar disorder. They can recognize when there is a problem in the realm of psychosis and are familiar with the medications used to treat it. Most family doctors will, however, defer further care to a psychiatrist. A psychiatrist is a medical doctor who has received additional training in the recognition and treatment of psychiatric disorders.

If it is the first onset of psychotic symptoms, the psychiatrist may ask for an MRI of the brain to rule out any causes such as tumors that are linked at times with unusual psychiatric symptoms. This risk is increased if the symptoms are unusual or if there are neurological symptoms.

COURSE

Fortunately, the symptoms are easily brought under control with proper medications. If the illness of schizophrenia remains untreated however, unusual fears and worries usually begin to preoccupy the person.

It is a challenge for a person suffering from schizophrenia to share their experiences or to give a logical description of what they are experiencing. They may grow silent and suspicious of others. Sometimes, they may perceive ill will from others. This can lead to unusual behaviors and agitation.

The course of schizophrenia is quite variable. Some individuals retain insight into the unusual nature of their experiences while others become enmeshed in them to a degree that they lose insight. They may feel that their unusual beliefs and delusions are true. Some may perceive their experiences to be a gift from God and may develop secondary messianic delusions.

At times, they may ascribe their unusual experiences to malevolent acts of government agencies or other individuals that want to harm them.

Sometimes the different delusions may link to each other in a systematized manner. Each delusion, in a sense, may reinforce the other. Such enmeshed and systematized delusions can be more resistant to treatment but do decrease with medications.

This web of fear that the illness weaves can lead many to cut off contact with others. Sometimes family members that want to help them may become woven into their delusional belief system as agents of a hostile world.

In schizoaffective disorder, in addition to the above, there are mood symptoms related to either depression or mania.

In the acute illness, it is hard to hold down a job or carry out some of the other roles that are second nature to most other people.

This illness affects the person in the prime of their life and loss of functioning may be very demoralizing. Depression symptoms can develop. It is important to offer the person a great deal of support and get help for the symptoms of depression as early as possible. Despair combined with a distorted reality can be a terrible burden.

The person with schizophrenia may believe that others can read their thoughts or take out their thoughts. In fact, this is not an unusual symptom. These particular symptoms are called delusions of thought insertion or thought withdrawal.

They may have a hard time explaining their experience. The more the person tries to share his or her concerns with others the more he or she may be met with surprised looks and concern about the strangeness of their symptoms and beliefs.

The net result, often, is that the ill person becomes secretive, isolative and afraid to share their private ideas and thoughts with others. Their world begins to get smaller, and they can begin to isolate themselves.

One of the symptoms of schizophrenia and schizoaffective disorder is avolition or lack of will to do things. They may thus neglect to take care of their basic hygiene needs or to tidy up around their room. Their surroundings may, therefore, become increasingly slovenly and disheveled. This may be reflected in their physical appearance as well.

At times, they can seem frozen in place in a condition called catatonia. Often this is related to their altered thought processes, which may become circuitous and ambivalent. Ambivalence is having equal feelings for and against an action. The person wants to do something but gets caught up in a see-saw of opposing desires and motives and never quite finishes what they began to do. It seems as if the person can not make up their mind. It can be a simple decision such as getting up to grab a newspaper or something. This ambivalence can make it difficult for any thought to reach a logical conclusion. While this internal tug of war is going on, the external activity may come to a stop and cease, giving the appearance of the person standing still and seemingly frozen in time.

It is an ironic situation because the external stillness belies the buzz of mental activity going on inside the person.

One of the unique symptoms of this condition is called waxy flexibility. In this, if a hand or arm is held up and let go, the person may continue to maintain the posture like a wax statue.

At other times, the internal struggle of the thought processes is manifested externally in the way of purposeless agitation. This is called catatonic agitation or agitated catatonia. It can become serious and lead to severe exhaustion, dehydration, muscle breakdown, renal shutdown, and even death.

Agitated catatonia or otherwise persistent catatonia is considered a psychiatric and a medical emergency and is one of the few conditions where electroconvulsive therapy (ECT) can be lifesaving. The first line of treatment, however, is often an injection of a medication called lorazepam in the dose of 2 to 3 mg. The medication dose may have to be repeated every few hours. If this does not work, a single dose of ECT can terminate the catatonic state described above.

With treatment, the person can begin to feel less distressed due to a decrease in the psychotic symptoms. This can occur in a matter of a week to ten days. The depressive symptoms can also improve in a matter of 3 to 4 weeks and sometimes sooner when antidepressant medications are offered.

Ask the doctor about any side effects and ask him to prescribe something to prevent the side effects. The improvement will continue for the next six to eight weeks. Continued treatment has the potential to remove many of the distortions and delusions.

Consistent compliance with medication and other prescribed treatments becomes the key to a full recovery. The willingness to try medication is essential to getting better. There are no other treatments that are effective for the treatment of hallucinations and delusions of schizophrenia.

If you are a family member, the best thing you can do is to encourage your loved one to take their medications and ensure that they get to their appointments with the doctor.

ARE THERE ANY LAB TESTS FOR SCHIZOPHRENIA?

There is no diagnostic lab test for schizophrenia. Some genes have been implicated but at this time there is no specific genetic scan for diagnosing schizophrenia. Certain labs may be ordered, however, to rule out medical illnesses that can produce psychotic symptoms.

How is the diagnosis of schizophrenia made?

The diagnosis of schizophrenia is made on the basis of the patient history, the diagnostic interview, and other observations. Certain labs may be ordered to rule out medical conditions or substance abuse issues. This is because certain medical conditions and substances can cause psychotic symptoms as well.

Is a family psychiatric history always present in someone with schizophrenia?

Often there is a family history of mental illness of a psychotic nature but this is not always the case. Schizophrenia or schizoaffective disorder can occur in someone without a family history of mental illness.

WHAT IS THE WORKUP FOR SCHIZOPHRENIA?

A psychiatrist has to consider a wide range of medical conditions before determining the symptoms to be due to schizophrenia.

The workup for schizophrenia is usually a combination of one or more of the following steps:

A. The taking of a careful history from the patient

B. A collateral history from family or friends

C. A medical history and review of symptoms

D. A physical examination

E. An EKG in some cases, depending on medical history

F. The following laboratory tests may be ordered:

- Urinalysis (UA)

- Urine Drug Screen (UDS)

- Urine pregnancy test in women of childbearing age

- Complete Blood Count (CBC)

- CMP (Comprehensive Metabolic Profile)

- This checks electrolytes, kidney function tests, calcium, phosphorus levels, bilirubin level and liver enzymes

- Lyme Antibody Titer

- ANA (Antinuclear Antibody Test) to rule out Systemic Lupus Erythematosus (SLE)

- RPR to rule out syphilis

- CT scan or MRI of the brain is indicated for unusual neurological or psychiatric symptoms. Some prefer this in all cases of first-time psychosis and the late-life onset of psychosis or mood disturbance

- HIV antibody test if indicated

- Serum ceruloplasmin test if copper metabolism problems are suspected

- 24-hour urine Porphyrin levels if indicated by family history and unusual color of urine

- Serum and urine heavy metal levels if indicated: If the patient has been exposed to heavy metals. This may occur in those who are employed in the mining industries

Unusual psychiatric symptoms such as visual, tactile or olfactory hallucinations always require a more detailed look for medical causes of such symptoms.

Illicit drug use can commonly cause psychotic symptoms. The presence of a positive urine drug screen and associated psychotic symptoms does not, however, always rule out a coexisting schizophrenia or schizoaffective disorder.

WHAT IS THE RATIONALE FOR SOME OF THE TESTS ORDERED FOR THE WORKUP OF SCHIZOPHRENIA?

The rationale for some of these tests is as follows.

1. CBC (Complete Blood Count)

This test can help in ruling out anemia and other blood-related illnesses. Anemia can have many causes due to different pathologies. If anemia exists, further tests can clarify the specific cause. Blood loss can occur due to a tumor of the gastrointestinal tract that can send metastasis to the brain. Certain micronutrient deficiencies can cause anemia and sometimes these deficiencies may increase the vulnerability to mental illness.

2. CMP (Comprehensive Metabolic Profile)

This panel checks for levels of electrolytes, BUN (Blood Urea Nitrogen), creatinine, glucose, liver enzymes, and bilirubin. Abnormal values in one or more can indicate the presence of kidney disease, liver disease, or endocrinological problems such as diabetes or abnormalities of the parathyroid glands. These medical diseases can have psychiatric repercussions.

3. TSH (Thyroid Stimulating Hormone)

This hormone is suppressed if the level of thyroid hormone is high and is elevated if the thyroid hormone levels are low. Thyroid abnormalities are can be associated with various psychiatric symptoms, hence this is a useful test to have. Some doctors will also add an FT4 (Free Thyroxine Level) to assess directly the level of circulating thyroid hormone.

4. RPR (Rapid Plasma Reagin)

This screening test helps to rule out an infection in the past or currently with syphilis. It interacts with any antibodies from a previous syphilis infection. Untreated syphilis can affect the brain and produce psychiatric symptoms. VDRL is another similar test to rule out syphilis. If the RPR or the VDRL is positive, it must be confirmed by another test called the fluorescent treponemal antibody test or the (FTA-ABS).

5. UA (Urinalysis)

This test can detect some medical problems such as untreated diabetes, kidney disease, liver disease, certain metabolic disorders, kidney stones, or infection of the urinary tract.

6. UDS (Urine Drug Screen)

This test is important to rule out psychotic symptoms that may be caused by various drugs of abuse such as amphetamines, phencyclidine, or the various hallucinogens.

7. Serum or Urine HcG

To rule out pregnancy

8. Brain-Imaging Scans

A CT scan or an MRI scan can help in ruling out any disease of the brain such as a tumor or stroke. This is especially relevant when psychiatric symptoms first present themselves late in life after age 40.

9. EEG (Electroencephalogram)

This is a recording made of the electrical activity of the brain. It is usually manifested as waves of different frequencies and shapes. It is a painless procedure. Various electrodes are placed on the surface of the different areas of the scalp to detect brain waves in different regions. If there are slow waves in a particular area of the brain, it may indicate brain pathology and malfunction in the underlying region of the brain.

In summary, an EEG is helpful in the following ways:

a) In epilepsy, rapid, spiking waves are seen

b) In tumors or strokes, slow waves may be detected from the area involved

c) In narcolepsy and petit mal epilepsy, unique diagnostic patterns are present

d) Diffuse, slow waves may be detected in generalized brain pathology from any cause. More specific tests can be ordered if such findings are noted

10. Lyme antibody:

Lyme disease can affect the central nervous system and produce unusual symptoms.

11. ANA antibody test

This can help rule out systemic lupus erythematosus or "lupus". This disease, or its treatment with steroids, can produce unusual psychiatric symptoms.

WHY IS IT IMPORTANT TO RULE OUT MEDICAL CAUSES?

It is important because medical problems can sometimes cause symptoms such as hallucinations and unusual thinking that is manifested by paranoia and delusional beliefs. To best treat these symptoms, the underlying medical condition requires treatment. Many times, the treatment of the underlying medical disorder may resolve the psychiatric difficulties.

Once the medical condition is treated, it may be possible to taper and discontinue the psychiatric medications.

While waiting for a medical workup, antipsychotic medications, and other psychiatric medications, are helpful in controlling symptoms <u>even if there is an associated medical condition.</u>

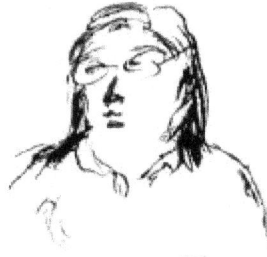

Differential Diagnosis in Schizophrenia

Schizoaffective Disorder
Bipolar Disorder with psychosis
Major Depression with psychosis
Drug Induced Psychosis
Medical Disorder related psychosis

WHAT CAUSES SCHIZOPHRENIA AND SCHIZOAFFECTIVE DISORDER?

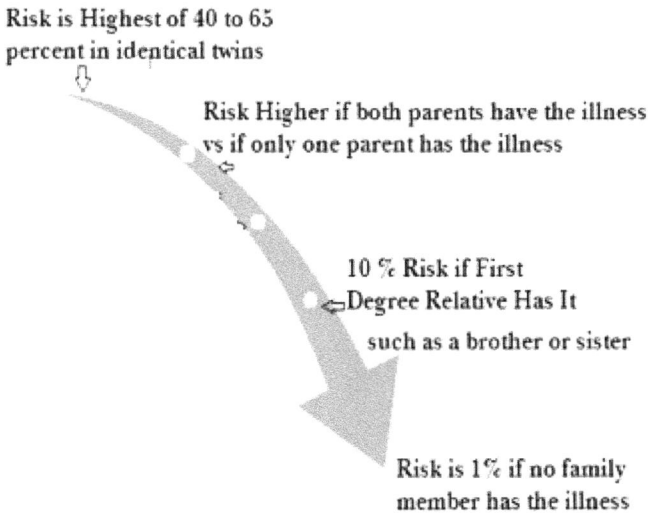

Risk is Highest of 40 to 65 percent in identical twins

Risk Higher if both parents have the illness vs if only one parent has the illness

10 % Risk if First Degree Relative Has It such as a brother or sister

Risk is 1% if no family member has the illness

Lower the Genetic Loading, Lower is the Risk for Schizophrenia and Schizoaffective Disorder

Many factors cause these illnesses. The cause is therefore listed as being multifactorial.

This assertion makes sense on an intuitive level as well. If the cause of these illnesses were one neurochemical or one gene gone awry, scientists would have possibly found the "magic bullet" to remedy that cause. The reality, however, is that a multifaceted approach is necessary for treatment of the illness that includes biological, social and psychological interventions. This approach best addresses the multifactorial causation of the illness.

Regarding the genetic causes of schizophrenia, we do not know the specific cause but do know for certain that there seems to be a large genetic contribution.

This is borne out by family studies where rates of schizophrenia are studied in family members of individuals diagnosed with schizophrenia.

According to these studies that are illustrated in the upside down arrow in the previous diagram, the rates of concordance (people sharing an illness) are highest in identical twins that have the identical set of genes. And it goes down from there. If one parent has it, the risk of a child having it is about 14 percent, and if two parents have it, it is about 42 percent. If a brother or sister has it, the rate is about 10 percent. In the normal population, with no other family member having the illness, the rate is about 1 percent.

There is a silver lining here, however. The fact that about 50 percent of identical twins don't have the illness while about half do indicates that the right environment can have a protective role even when the genes are identical in two individuals. The individual with the right environmental factors may escape the illness while the other one develops the symptoms. We will touch upon this a bit later as well.

What we do know is that there seems to be some genetic contribution as the incidence of schizophrenia is higher in other family members. The environment also seems to play a role as biologically identical twins with the same set of genes sometimes differ in the emergence of the illness if their environments are different. One twin might have the illness while the other twin brought up in a different environment may not.

The emergence of schizophrenia is truly a product of the interplay between both nature and nurture.

The genes interact in a unique way with environmental factors to cause abnormal neurochemistry. The full effect of the disordered neurochemistry is only manifest once the brain has matured at around age 21.

For this reason, the onset of the illness is typically seen in the early twenties. For a long time now, an infectious agent such as the influenza virus or other infectious agents has been suspected to be the key environmental trigger for schizophrenia.

This conclusion was based on the fact that there is seasonality in the birth months for individuals that suffer from schizophrenia. This seems to correlate with the fact that there is seasonality to the flu virus as well. This theory has not been conclusively proven, neither has it been disproven.

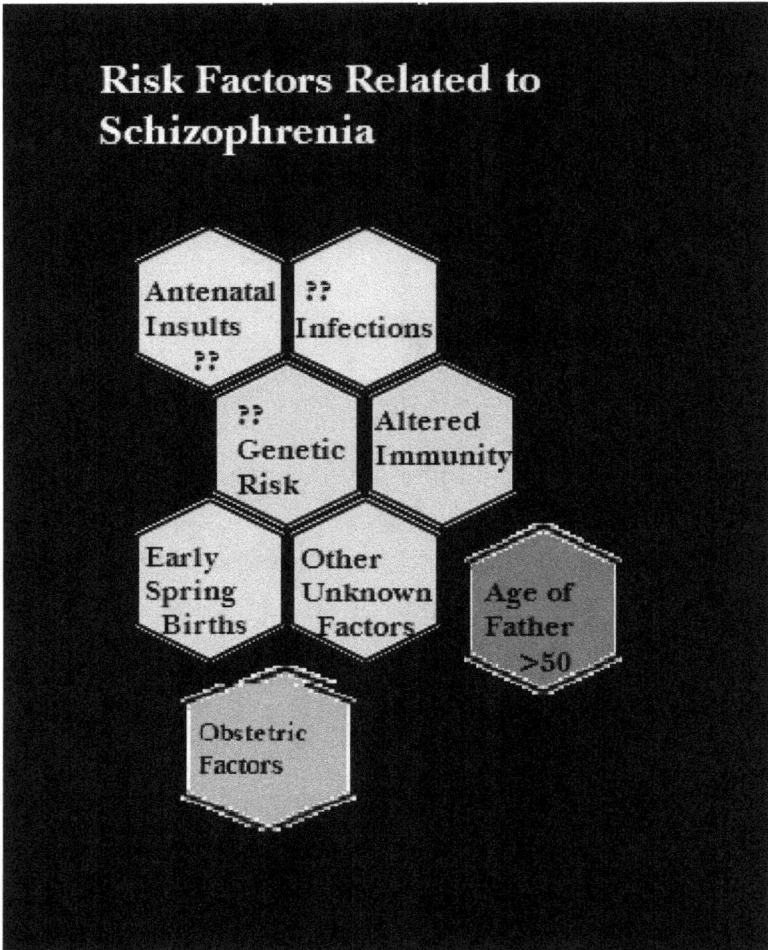

Risk Factors Related to Schizophrenia

- Antenatal Insults ??
- ?? Infections
- ?? Genetic Risk
- Altered Immunity
- Early Spring Births
- Other Unknown Factors
- Age of Father >50
- Obstetric Factors

The best guess is that exposure to infections probably does have a role. It is likely that certain infections during a vulnerable period of brain development may affect the future course of neural migration and development in the young brain. After the brain has developed, the neurodevelopment is unlikely to be affected any further by infections in a similar way. Hence, late-onset schizophrenia is very rare and if such symptoms appear, they always call for a vigorous search to rule out medical disease. In essence, schizophrenia appears to be a neurodevelopmental disorder that become manifest at the full maturation of the brain around age 21 and sometimes sooner.

IS THERE A GENE THAT CAUSES SCHIZOPHRENIA?

Chromosome 22 has been implicated in some studies. This, however, has not been noted to be a consistent finding. It is more likely that multiple genes located on multiple chromosomes are related to the expression of schizophrenia.

The genes control many aspects of neural development and activation of neurochemical events. They may be triggered in different ways by a combination of environmental stressors such as infections, illnesses, or trauma related to physical or emotional abuse.

The role of certain genes appears to be linked in the causation of schizophrenia. These genes seem to be valuable. While they are associated with the production of the illness of schizophrenia, under the right circumstances they can also produce brilliant thinkers and scientists. This is well evidenced by the presence of schizophrenia in close family members of several Nobel laureates.

The age of the father also seems to be a factor. In fathers over age 50, the risk for schizophrenia in the offspring is about three times higher than a father in his twenties or thirties. The exact mechanism for this is not clear yet but is worthy of further study.

Even the stress level of the mother in the first months of her pregnancy has been correlated with a higher incidence of schizophrenia in the offspring. For example, if there has been a significant stressor during the first month of the pregnancy with the mother, such as the death of a loved one, or another significant setback, the risk of developing schizophrenia in the child may be slightly higher.

Emotions are powerful things. It is important that we take care of our emotions as if they were a well-tended garden. To ignore the sanctity of our emotions is to invite the weeds of mental illness to sprout and choke out what is good in our life.

CAN SOME OF THE "GENETIC INFLUENCE" BE THE RESULT OF LEARNED CHILD REARING BEHAVIORS THAT ARE PASSED FROM ONE GENERATION TO THE NEXT?

Some families are dysfunctional in the way that they raise their children.

Sometimes the parents can be highly intelligent and lead an intellectual existence that is not swayed by normal day to day emotional upheavals. The parents may treat the child as a miniature adult and not provide the love, play and warmth that is needed for healthy emotional development of the child.

A lack of strong reciprocity of emotions can create an ambivalent emotional climate that is interpreted by the child as a rejecting climate. The cold and aloof parent that neither accepts or rejects, that alternates rejection and then acceptance without a predictable pattern, is starving the child of emotional nurturance that is needed for healthy brain development in the first twenty-one years of its life. The rate of growth is the greatest in the first ten years but continues till the later years.

The child may grow into a dysfunctional or semifunctional adult who is never able to truly love with passion or intensity and rears his or her own children in a similar manner. The cycle can thus be perpetuated from generation to generation. The Dr. Spock admonitions about letting children cry themselves to sleep in their own room must have also created an aloof and emotionally sterile climate for those children. The parents must have felt self-righteous because it was endorsed by the "scientific" opinion of the medical community. Such advice probably did more harm than any good, but the practice persists.

At a higher level, the greater parent, the parens patriae, the government, has totally abandoned all responsibility for the healthy growth of families. Many middle-class families have to struggle with both parents juggling multiple jobs to make ends meet. The rates of divorce are at an all-time high. The family leave act is still not the law of the land when a young woman becomes a mother. Many states require the mother to return to work within a few weeks and leave the rearing of her child to others.

Individuals raised in such an environment, unless they understand and overcome the obstacles, are likely to repeat this with their own children. Hence the "genetic influence" may not be entirely genetic but learned toxic behavior that is passed from generation to generation leading to higher rates of mental illness in some families. This learned behavior appears to be a real factor that is overlooked.

IS THERE A WAY TO GET A GENETIC TEST FOR SCHIZOPHRENIA OR SCHIZOAFFECTIVE DISORDER?

There are some companies that offer genome scans based on saliva samples to predict the genetic risk for various diseases. At this time, however, such "genome scans" are unlikely to provide useful information about the risk of developing a mental disorder like schizophrenia or schizoaffective disorder.

This is because the cause of schizophrenia or schizoaffective disorder has not been localized to one gene. It probably has a polygenetic contribution and the genes seem to be expressed under certain environmental triggers that are prone to differ in the life circumstances of every human being.

Many environmental factors may be involved, such as exposure to viruses or malnutrition before birth, problems during childbirth and early childhood, and other perhaps yet unknown factors.

The final expression of the illness is in an altered neurochemistry in the brain cells and the synapses between brain cells where they communicate with each other via neurochemicals such as dopamine, norepinephrine, serotonin and others.

These serve to activate or inhibit different receptors on the cells causing a further cascade of neurochemical events. The chances for misfiring and miscommunication are vast. It is a miracle that the brain functions remarkably well in so many individuals. By the same token, the brains of every human being, and even identical twins are different from each other.

PIONEERS OF SCHIZOPHRENIA RECOGNITION

In 1887, Emile Kraepelin, a great German psychiatrist, observed and studied mental illness in large mental health hospitals for the chronically ill. He recognized that some of these patients had a decline in function paralleling the way in which a person with dementia declines in function.

Since these individuals were of a relatively young age, he called it Dementia Praecox. This illness is now called schizophrenia today. He further classified the illness into different subtypes. The subtypes he used were as follows:

1. Disorganized type

2. Catatonic type

3. Paranoid type

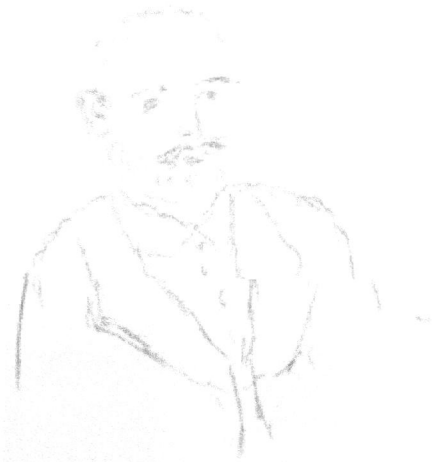

Dr. Emile Kraeplin
Early German
Psychiatrist 1887

He was an observant man, and his classification system has stood the test of time with minor modifications. The details of these subtypes will be discussed later.

In 1911, Paul Eugen Bleuler, a Swiss psychiatrist, coined the actual term schizophrenia. Schizo means split and phrenia means mind. It literally means, "split mind". Some individuals are liable to misinterpret this as a condition of "split personality".

"Split personality", however, is a rare and totally different condition. Split personality is usually related to traumatic emotional events and overwhelming threat to the physical integrity of the individual. It is a way of sealing deep-seated fears in order to go on with the rest of one's life.

It has little to do with schizophrenia or schizoaffective disorder. The condition will be explained in some more detail later.

Dr. Bleuler, who coined the word schizophrenia, was also the first to classify symptoms of schizophrenia into the categories of positive symptoms and negative symptoms. This classification system is still valid today and often used by psychiatrists to describe the progress made by a patient.

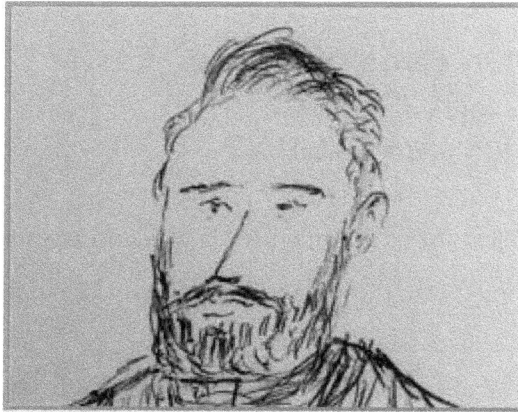

**Dr. Paul Eugen Bleuler
In 1911 coined the word
Schizophrenia**

Positive and Negative Symptoms

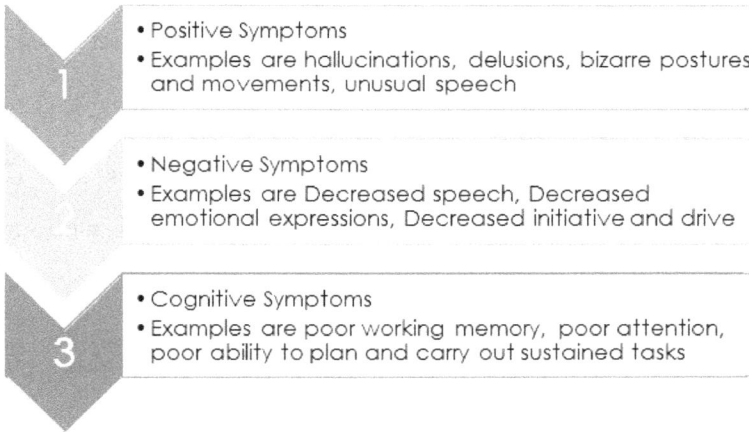

- **1**
  - Positive Symptoms
  - Examples are hallucinations, delusions, bizarre postures and movements, unusual speech

- **2**
  - Negative Symptoms
  - Examples are Decreased speech, Decreased emotional expressions, Decreased initiative and drive

- **3**
  - Cognitive Symptoms
  - Examples are poor working memory, poor attention, poor ability to plan and carry out sustained tasks

Negative symptoms were defined as deficits in the functioning of the individual. These were functions that the patients with schizophrenia had apparently lost. For example, a normal person will usually initiate conversation, to seek contact with others, and may initiate some purposeful activity or other. This may be lacking to a remarkable degree in schizophrenia.

This lack of initiative was classified by Dr. Bleuler as a negative symptom he called avolition. Avolition was defined as the lack of will (to initiate things). Others have termed the same condition abulia or a lack of drive. Alogia is a related negative symptom having to do with a deficit of speech output. This deficit is not simply due to the person being anxious or shy but is an inherent symptom of schizophrenia.

The positive symptoms that Bleuler described, on the other hand, were new, additional features that emerged in the person with schizophrenia. These features are not normally found in individuals without schizophrenia.

For example, a person with schizophrenia may hear voices. This is an added feature that is not present in ordinary persons without schizophrenia.

Since it is an added feature, it is called a positive symptom although there is nothing positive about it.

These "positive symptoms", such as hallucinations, are some of the most distressful symptoms of schizophrenia.

Similarly, delusions or fixed false beliefs are another "positive symptom" that is absent in the experience of most individuals.

WHAT ARE THE COMMON HALLUCINATIONS AND DELUSIONS IN SCHIZOPHRENIA AND SCHIZOAFFECTIVE DISORDER?

A common hallucination is a voice that a person hears that no one else hears. Sometimes there may be more than one voice at the same time. The voice may keep up a running commentary on everything that the person is doing or that is going on in a person's life.

The voice is usually critical, condescending and annoying, although comforting voices are also reported sometimes. The voice at different times may give advice, cajole, or threaten a person. They sometimes may command a person to carry out some action. They may threaten the person with dire consequences if the person does not carry out the action.

A Voice That Won't Go Away

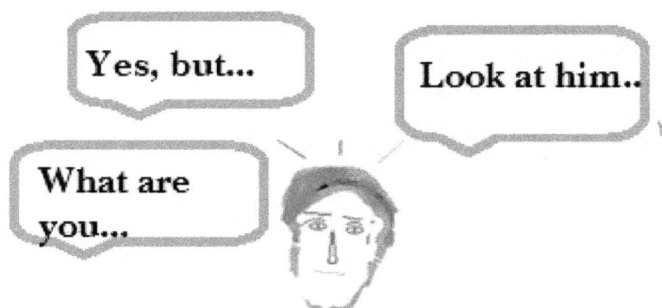

A constant stream of a voice or voices may bother the person with schizophrenia. The voice may criticize him, call him names, yell at him, and threaten him. Sometimes two voices may comment on what the person is doing. The person wants them to stop but is not able to make the voice go away.

The actions the voices ask the person to do can be simple, such as placing a certain article in a certain way, or they may ask the person to perform dangerous actions towards themselves or others. Most individuals learn to ignore the voices and do not always act on them even if they are threatened. These hallucinations that command a person to do something are called command hallucinations and are taken very seriously by clinicians.

If command hallucinations occur, an intervention from a psychiatrist should be sought as early as possible. This may sometimes necessitate admission to a psychiatric unit where safety can be ensured, and the symptoms can be brought under control through treatment with medications.

WHAT IS THE OUTLOOK FOR SOMEONE DIAGNOSED WITH SCHIZOPHRENIA?

It is generally good as treatment can decrease many of the symptoms within one to two weeks. Further improvement and decrease of symptoms continues over the next few weeks. With treatment, a person can again pursue their life goals that may have been interrupted. It is important to emphasize this positive outlook to prevent demoralization or depression that can emerge when the symptoms first appear. The symptoms can be very annoying and disconcerting and the person may for the first time feel out of control.

Treating doctors have some very effective medications at their disposal that can bring predictable and reliable relief of symptoms. Schizophrenia no longer needs to be an illness that causes fear or despair.

Many people who have the disorder learn to ignore their voices. Infrequently, some even find comfort from the voices if they are encouraging or soothing. Some prominent people have achieved success despite the handicaps imposed by their illness.

GOOD HABITS THAT PREVENT RELAPSE

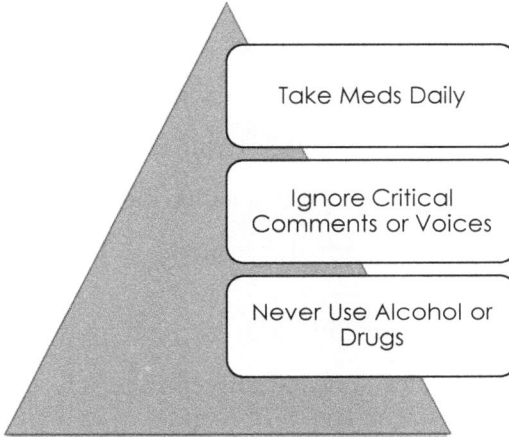

Take Meds Daily

Ignore Critical Comments or Voices

Never Use Alcohol or Drugs

HOW CAN PARANOIA LEAD TO PROBLMS?

Paranoia can cause problms when the person begins acting on their fears and mistaken notions. For example, the individual may feel that others are talking about him on the TV or in the newspapers. The person may interpret simple routine acts in the environment as a person talking to another person as having something to do with him. These are called referential delusions.

These can be very distressful to the person and may make them feel that they are under constant surveillance. They may try to get away or flee from their location so that others stop referring to them and the media stop broadcasting about them. At other times, they may become agitated and threatening towards their perceived persecutors.

Such agitation or assaultive behaviors may lead to an arrest or incarceration. With time, it may become harder and more difficult for them to trust anyone.

The individual in such a situation should be offered support and yet given enough space to allow them to feel comfortable. Medical and psychiatric assistance should be sought as soon as possible. Educational material providing knowledge about their symptoms and treatment can be helpful in the long run. Knowing that their symptoms are caused by a treatable illness that has a name can be reassuring at some level.

Supportive family members and friends can be crucial at this juncture.

It is important to provide hope to the individual and let the person know that their symptoms are treatable. They should be told that the symptoms can go into a lasting remission and that they need not feel hopeless or overwhelmed.

REMEMBER: ASKING FOR HELP IS OK

It may be difficult, but it is helpful to confide in a trusted friend or family member. That family member should be comforting to them and should not be unduly alarmed. Individuals with schizophrenia are not generally dangerous, and the illness does not carry the dire prognosis that it once did.

The family member and the individual should seek help from a psychiatrist or through their local doctor as soon as possible. If the issues are emergent, it is perfectly OK to call 911 or go to an emergency room. Early treatment and supportive care lead to a better outcome for those who suffer from schizophrenia.

WHAT IS A PERSONALITY DISORDER?

It is relevant to talk about personality disorders in the discussion of schizophrenia as they can sometimes be confused with psychotic illness. A personality disorder is a behavioral pattern that causes difficulties in the ability to get along with others. The relationships of individuals with personality disorder always suffer in one way or another.

Many individuals with a personality disorder therefore have a higher frequency of divorce problems in their personal life and occupational problems in their public life.

Some individuals with antisocial personality disorder, narcissistic personality disorder, or a borderline personality disorder may feel entitled and above the normal rules and constraints of society. They may thus breach the law of the land and run into legal problems of one kind or another.

WHAT ARE SOME PERSONALITY DISORDERS THAT MAY BE CONFUSED WITH PSYCHOTIC ILLNESS?

Individuals with the following personality disorders may appear unusual in their mannerisms and behaviors and suspicion may arise about their state of mind, i.e. whether they suffer from a psychotic illness such as schizophrenia or schizoaffective disorder.

Let us review these and look at the distinguishing features.

1. Schizotypal Personality Disorder: This type of personality disorder is marked by unusual behaviors and manners of attire, dress and manner. These individuals are not psychotic but just have a peculiar way of relating and expressing themselves. They may at times be perceived as being mentally ill. They may experience very transient states of psychosis but are generally lucid, logical and in touch with reality.

2. Schizoid Personality Disorder: Individuals with this personality disorder prefer to be alone and shun the company of others. They are not distressed by their self-imposed isolation and prefer this as their mode of existence. They do not suffer from hallucinations or delusions and are normal in other ways.

3. Paranoid Personality Disorder: This type of individual tends to misperceive the actions of others as hostile or exploitative.

They may pursue litigation as a means to address the wrong they perceive to have occurred to them. They, at times, may appear to be paranoid and delusional, but there is often some basis to their grievance. They can be convinced out of some mistaken notions in contrast to the person that is truly delusional. Furthermore, they do not have hallucinations and, as mentioned, are not delusional. They are often intelligent and tend to overanalyze matters, giving undue weight to details that escape the notice of others. Their defining attitude is to verify and then trust rather than trust and verify.

4. Individuals with PTSD: These individuals may also prefer isolation and may be distrustful of others due to their past traumas or abuse. They are not psychotic and are able to trust certain individuals that they have faith in. Many movies depict this feature of the PTSD veterans accurately. An example of this is the movie First Blood wherein the veteran Rambo, afflicted by PTSD, only trusts his commanding officer, Col. Sam Trautman.

5. Borderline Personality Disorder: Individuals with this personality disorder may have transient psychotic episodes during a period of high stress but generally have intact reality testing. Their relationships tend to vacillate from overvaluation to devaluation and the rush to negative judgment may make them appear irrational. They, however, lack the other persisting dysfunctions associated with

schizoaffective disorder or schizophrenia such as persisting hallucinations or delusions. Very transient psychotic episodes may be experienced in individuals with borderline personality disorder when they are under extreme stress.

6. Personality-disordered individuals who are intoxicated: Individuals with certain personality disorders such as antisocial personality disorder, borderline personality disorder or a narcissistic personality disorder may abuse certain drugs and have a general sense of entitlement and self-centeredness. The drug use may exacerbate grandiosity and produce manic or psychotic symptoms. These symptoms are transient and wear off with sobriety.

WHAT ABOUT SOME INDIVIDUALS THAT BELIEVE SCHIZOPHRENIA IS NOT A REAL ILLNESS?

Schizophrenia is a real illness and those who say it is not are plain wrong. It is not the mere expression of existential angst by an individual caught up in the web of "an insane society".

As charming and as appealing as these theories appear to be, the fact is that schizophrenia and schizoaffective disorder are disabling and take a severe toll on the person and society.

They carry the burden of severe and specific symptoms and are reliably treated with specific medications. A factitious illness would not respond to any medication because it does not exist. There is evidence of gross anatomical changes and subtle neurochemical changes and metabolic abnormalities in the brain of individuals affected by schizophrenia. On a practical level, the illness is very real to the person who suffers from it and to his family and friends who see him or her struggle with it.

HOW COMMON IS SUBSTANCE ABUSE IN INDIVIDUALS WITH SCHIZOPHRENIA AND SCHIZOAFFECTIVE DISORDER AND HOW DOES IT COMPLICATE THEIR LIVES?

Screening of Individuals with Substance Abuse Problems and Psychosis

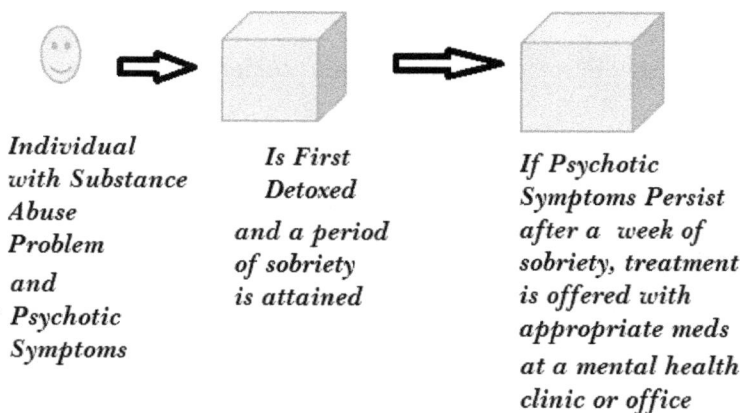

Individual with Substance Abuse Problem and Psychotic Symptoms

Is First Detoxed and a period of sobriety is attained

If Psychotic Symptoms Persist after a week of sobriety, treatment is offered with appropriate meds at a mental health clinic or office

The prevalence of substance use among patients with schizophrenia and schizoaffective disorder varies in different countries and locations. In the urban areas of the United States, the prevalence rates of substance and alcohol abuse can be as high as 50%. It often complicates the lives of individuals with mental illness, sometimes leading to homelessness and rough existence on the streets.

These individuals in their homeless state are often victimized by drug dealers or other antisocial elements. At other times, they may themselves resort to criminal activities to provide for food and other basic needs. Such unlawful behaviors, even if minor, can lead to a trip to the local jail and sometimes to prisons for more serious crimes.

Street drugs and alcohol invariably worsen the symptoms of psychosis, depression or mania for all patients. The stimulant drugs and PCP can produce a drug-induced psychotic episode that can be hard to distinguish from the primary illness of schizophrenia or schizoaffective disorder.

Getting help is not always easy. Many community centers will not accept a patient for services if they are actively using drugs. Although the underlying reason may be the underfunding of the community mental health center, the ostensible reason for such a cop out is the excuse that drug-induced psychosis cannot be distinguished from a real psychotic illness while the patient is using the drugs.

Many skilled clinicians, however, can make the distinction as the episodes of psychosis in drug-induced states are circumscribed and have a different quality to them, and there is a return to normal level of functioning with sobriety.

Some centers are more understanding and do offer a detoxification facility to help the individual attain sobriety and get further mental health help as needed.

HOW FREQUENT IS THE RATE OF SMOKING IN INDIVIDUALS WITH SCHIZOPHRENIA?

There is a higher rate of smoking in patients that suffer from schizophrenia and other major mental disorders. A rate as high as 80% has been cited in some studies. This contributes to a significant increase in health problems for some individuals. A less well-known fact is that smoking can lower the levels of the medications, rendering them less effective than they would otherwise be. When a patient gives up smoking, their physical and mental health tends to improve. Smoking cessation, therefore, is an effort worth making.

HOW DOES ONE DIFFERENTIATE THE DIFFERENT TYPES OF PSYCHOTIC DISORDERS FROM SCHIZOPHRENIA?

By definition, schizophrenia is an illness marked by hallucinations or delusions that that have lasted for more than six months. These symptoms also cause dysfunction. This is in the form of problems with the person's ability to function at home, at school, at work or in other settings. There are distinctive positive and negative symptoms and unique features such as loosening of associations.

In contrast, a brief psychotic disorder is a psychosis that lasts from 1 to 30 days. There is a loss of touch with reality by definition. The constellation of psychotic symptoms can vary.

Schizophreniform disorder is a psychotic illness that lasts for less than six months and is self-limiting. It is diagnosed when the duration of illness is greater than one month but less than six months. The symptoms can look like schizophrenia.

Schizoaffective disorder is diagnosed when prominent mood symptoms, either depression or mania, coexist and the criteria for schizophrenia are also met.

Individuals with a delusional disorder have a circumscribed belief about some issue. The delusion may be within the normal range of experiences that other people share such as being swindled or being cheated upon by a spouse. Delusions may also be bizarre such as the belief that the person is from another planet. Delusional beliefs are circumscribed and may not be apparent unless the person is observed over a period of time. The person with a delusional disorder may continue to function normally otherwise in other areas of their life except for the area that they are delusional about.

Bipolar disorder can be associated with severe mania or severe depression. Severe mania can be associated with grandiose delusions of great power or abilities. These delusions remit once the mania is controlled. Depression in the severe form can be associated with nihilistic delusions that the world has ended, and the person is dead. A unique delusional state associated with such nihilistic delusions is called Cotard syndrome. In this syndrome, the person is alive but feels that their insides have rotted and that they are dead or almost dead. They have a resigned attitude of despair and utter hopelessness. For rapid relief, ECT can be lifesaving. Treatment is otherwise with a combination of antidepressants and antipsychotics. The expected time course of response to treatment is four to six weeks. Sometimes, an earlier response to treatment may occur.

CHAPTER 3

THE ROLE OF FAMILY AND FRIENDS

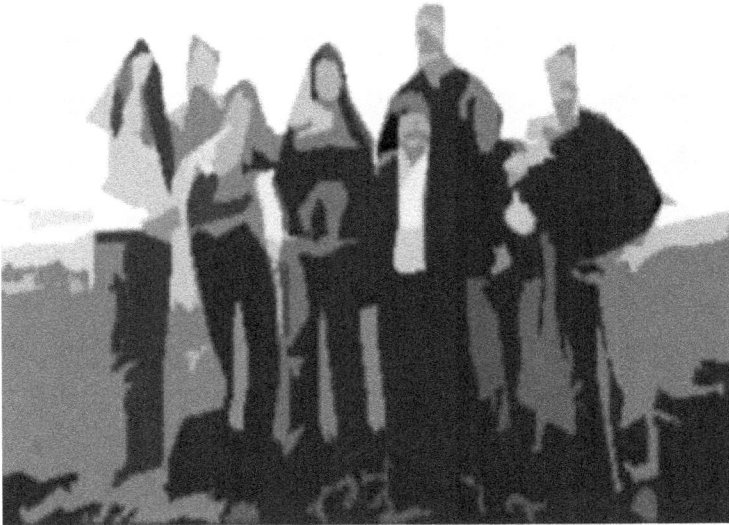

FAMILIES & FRIENDS ARE IMPORTANT

They can be helpful by

1. Encouraging the individual to take their medications and to go to their appointments.

2. By avoiding loud critical arguments with each other and with the person that suffers from schizophrenia or schizoaffective disorder.

HOW CAN FAMILIES AND FRIENDS BE HELPFUL?

Families and friends can help in some of the following ways:

1. Be respectful and polite. Let the person know in a polite manner if their behaviors are causing problems.

2. Always be their advocate and accompany them to their appointments when necessary.

3. If they have to go to the emergency room, try to accompany them and take the relevant medical records, insurance papers, a list of their current medications and other information that may be helpful.

4. Support the use of long-acting medications when available and discuss this with the individual and the doctor.

5. Remove any dangerous weapons or firearms from their vicinity to lower the risk of harm to them and others.

6. Remove alcohol from their vicinity and get help for them if they have any problems with alcohol or substance abuse.

7. Provide positive feedback for any gains made and also for efforts made towards recovery.

8. Provide unconditional positive regard for their humanity. Do not let them feel stigmatized and less as human beings.

9. Encourage compliance with medications and good health practices.

10. Encourage a tobacco-free lifestyle.

11. Encourage attendance at support groups and go to their NAMI meetings when you can. It will be greatly appreciated.

WHAT IS THE ROLE OF NAMI AND SELF-HELP GROUPS IN THE RECOVERY PROCESS?

NAMI stands for the national alliance on mental illness. This is a vanguard organization that advocates for individuals with mental illness. The NAMI website at https://www.nami.org/ provides information about local organizers and local self-help groups and other resources in the community.

Sometimes seeing another individual successfully overcome their schizophrenia symptoms can provide a big motivational boost for an individual who is struggling with their symptoms. Seeing others function at a high level can also relieve many other anxieties that they may have about their condition.

Being part of a larger organization such as NAMI also helps them to advocate as a group for the mental health treatment issues within the community. Participation in such self-help groups should be encouraged when they are available locally.

IF SOMEONE EXPERIENCES THE SYMPTOMS, WHAT SHOULD THEY DO?

It is important for them to confide in a friend or family member. That family member should comfort them and not be unduly alarmed. Schizophrenia does not carry the dire prognosis that it once did. They should seek help from their local doctor or emergency room if necessary.

Early treatment and supportive care are conducive to a better prognosis and outlook for the individual.

HOW DOES PSYCHOSIS EVOLVE OVER TIME?

This is a fascinating question and for one which we do not have precise answers. We don't know how subtle alterations in brain chemistry and receptors create hallucinations. We know even less about how erroneous beliefs are produced and how they consolidate and crystallize into unshakeable delusions that are impervious to all logic.

One can only make conjectures at possible mechanisms.

It is helpful to start with an understanding of the role of the human brain. The purpose of the brain is to keep us alive, ensure our safety and protect those we care about. For the brain to achieve this, it is always gathering information from many different sources and analyzing it to achieve the above-stated goals.

It is especially perceptive and sensitive to any dangers or threats in the environment. The more anxious and fearful the brain is, the more hungry it becomes for information.

The brain is a finely tuned instrument, elegantly designed for survival. It does this by analysis of incoming information.

When information is lacking, it uses logic, and leaps of logic, to make sense of a confusing world. It creates possible scenarios of threat or danger and then makes plans to ward off such potential dangers.

If high anxiety is generated by an ambivalent relationship or unpredictable behaviors of a parent or other caretaker, it does not help the situation. When strange hallucinations and voices emerge at the beginning of a psychotic illness, it produces a similar quandary and anxiety, leading to the brain working overtime to figure out answers for the unusual symptoms.

In a high-strung, anxious state, the brain is likely to distort incoming stimuli and misinterpret the information that it does gather.

Hallucinations generated by the unique neurochemistry of the schizophrenic brain create a reality that challenges the brain to come up with answers. As mentioned, the brain abhors the "I don't know" state. When a voice starts speaking, and no source is found, the brain seems to make up an answer if the I don't know state is prolonged.

This answer could be that God, the devil, aliens or their dead relative or some other entity are producing the voices. This assumption will generate the next set of questions such as why and how and for what purpose?

This can lead to the next set of tentative answers. Conspiratorial theories may arise and fall, and some may gel into delusional beliefs.

The person will then try to figure out how to deal with these voices. They may talk back to them timidly at first, and then in an angry way, and ask them to leave them alone. They may do this aloud in public and generate curiosity from onlookers, which further amplifies their anxiety and self-consciousness. This can amplify the ambiance of a noxious environment that much more.

Ambivalent relationships with no clear signs of approval or disapproval create a caldron wherein such delusions may form to provide a stable platform of thought, even if it is an erroneous one. It has been rightly postulated by psychoanalysts from the earliest days that the cold and aloof parents who provided basic support but no positive regard or support were key to generating schizophrenic states in their children. By the same token, the giving of inconsistent rewards and punishments generated the same atmosphere of suspense and unpredictability.

In the politically correct climate of modern-day psychiatry, the role of emotional climate in the home is minimized. This, however, overlooks an important aspect of causation that may be at play in some cases. These factors need to be considered and therapeutically addressed to facilitate the full recovery of the individual.

It may mean emancipation from toxic caregivers, the teaching of caregivers and creation of a stable, supportive and responsive environment that meets the emotional needs of the individual.

The key would be to provide a consistent and reliable group of people where the person is never in doubt about their ultimate acceptance and value acceptability within the group. Within this group, they would know that they are safe and can relax.

Such factors should be considered when making a treatment and rehabilitation plan for the individual.

DEVELOPMENT OF CATATONIC FEATURES:

The person in the acute phase of their illness may be so distracted by their hallucinations and the accompanying rationalizations, thoughts and developing delusions that they may begin to neglect basic acts of hygiene and self-care.

The person may be plunged into a state of intense ambivalence over minor matters. They may have conflicting ideas that alternate with one another on an endless loop that they cannot seem to get themselves out of. While they are preoccupied intensely with such a phenomenon, they may remain transfixed in one pose. The person is intensely self-aware during such states but is so transfixed by his mental phenomenon that he makes limited outside responses.

On recovery, they will describe vague feelings of paranoia and loss of control but often will not talk about the specific issues of concern. Once they are better, they seem to have some insight about the phenomenon.

During the catatonic state, the person seems to be on an autopilot of sorts. If their hand is placed in midair, they may passively submit and retain that pose. They may hold the position for a long time. This symptom is called the wax statue sign or the waxy flexibility sign. The person holds their pose like a wax statue. It is also called by the Latin term cerea flexibilitas.

Due to other cerebral functions being on autopilot, the patient may give automatic responses at other levels such as repetition of whatever is said, or echolalia, or copying whatever is done in front of them (echopraxia) or automatic resistance to any push or pull of their body, also called by the German term gegenhalten.

WHAT ARE SOME KEY TIPS TO KEEP IN MIND WHEN TALKING TO A PERSON ABOUT THEIR DELUSIONAL BELIEFS?

One should not argue with the patient about their delusions. These are very real to them even if they seem irrational and bizarre to you. It is important to listen to their concerns and express sympathy for the anxiety they may be feeling without directly arguing about the details of their concerns.

One may suggest that taking medications can sometimes help ease the anxiety symptoms and encourage a visit with a doctor.

If the patient is already prescribed medications then the family member or friend should encourage regular compliance with the medications.

If the medication is not helping or causing side effects that cause noncompliance then the family member or friend should speak with the doctor to help change the medication or add other medications to control any side effects.

In this way, by offering sympathy and support for the anxiety, you can continue to have a supportive relationship and encourage the individual to get help.

WHAT ARE SOME GENERAL GUIDELINES FOR FAMILIES AND FRIENDS OF THE INDIVIDUAL THAT SUFFERS FROM SCHIZOPHRENIA?

These are as follows:

Be an advocate for the person.

Be knowledgeable about the symptoms and signs.

Get in touch with a doctor early to adjust meds if you see signs of relapse.

Be supportive and do not speak loudly or engage in arguments.

Do not try to reason them out of their beliefs but express sympathy for their anxiety.

Check whether they are taking their medicine.

Ask if there are any side effects that are maybe bothering them.

Do not be too intrusive.

Do not try to analyze your loved ones and try to make pronouncements about their motives or reasons.

Such statements can be belittling and disqualify the suffering associated with the symptoms.

You may offer to discuss any recent losses or setbacks. The conversation can be initiated simply as, "I know some days can be stressful. How are you holding up? Do you want to talk about it?" This can help to decrease their stress level.

If they choose not to talk about it, respect their wishes.

If the individual shows signs of neglecting self-care or talks about harming themselves, take it seriously and contact their doctor for further advice. Hospitalization is advisable if the risk for self-harm or harm to others is high.

Remove guns whenever possible. Having guns around is a recipe for disaster.

Have a family member keep a watch on them until help can be obtained if they are in an acute crisis.

If you feel threatened, trust your instincts, allow the individual space, and keep safe.

Allow the professional authorities and staff to handle any dangerous behaviors but remain their advocate.

If the police are called, let the dispatcher know that the person suffers from a mental illness and indicate if the person is unarmed so that no lethal force is used.

If you are on the scene and know that the individual does not have a gun, let the police know and that he or she has a mental illness.

Some police jurisdictions provide training in mental health to their officers so that they are conversant with talking down the person and in avoiding unnecessary confrontations.

WHAT IS A TOXIC FAMILY MEMBER?

Most family members are loving, caring and deeply troubled by any illness in a family member.

However, there are toxic family members that can make a bad situation worse. A toxic family member is a parent, a spouse, a sibling or another relation that is manipulative and abusive to the person that is dependent, sick or physically challenged in some way.

The dependent person may be a child or an adult of any age that suffers from schizophrenia or another handicap.

Given the breadth of human behaviors, every clinician comes across some such parents, spouses and caretakers that are toxic to the patient they are trying to heal and make whole.

Dr. M Scott Peck writes eloquently of this in his book, *People of the Lie*.

A toxic person can be openly or covertly hostile, critical, and condescending. They may make snide and sly comments to undermine the integrity or the value of the person or try to tell them how they cannot do something even when the individual has shown that he or she can. They may belittle by saying how they always fail etc. or bring up any past setbacks as reminders of their ineptness.

Some individuals such as this may be acting out of their own insecurities and anxieties. They often do these things to meet some unconscious need of their own to feel superior. The toxic person often possesses an abundance of narcissistic and/or antisocial traits.

The individual with toxic behaviors can sometimes change their ways after being called on it. On the other hand, they may have gotten so used to not being questioned and having things go their way that they fail to realize that anything is amiss or wrong. They may even challenge the clinician and demand a change of clinician when their narcissistic sense of entitlement to abuse is challenged.

Toxic individuals that are amenable to learning can benefit from training and education. Improvement is especially likely if legal consequences are a possibility due to persisting abusive behaviors.

If they are not willing to change themselves, getting the individual with schizophrenia away from such a toxic person can be one of the first steps towards improving the mental health of the patient.

In some cases, the child protective services or adult protective services may need to be called to secure the welfare of the sick individual.

WHAT ARE SOME STEPS THE FAMILY CAN TAKE WHEN THIS ILLNESS IS DIAGNOSED IN A FAMILY MEMBER?

It is important to gather family members in a meeting. The head of the family should tell everyone about the facts of the illness. He should indicate that the family needs to support the individual and that it is treatable.

It may be necessary to explain that the individual may appear sloppy and unmotivated to take care of cleaning around him or herself. They may also appear neglectful of their appearance and attention to hygiene and grooming may be affected.

It should be explained that avolition (lack of will) is a feature of the illness and that it does not indicate that the person is lazy or trying to pass on work to others. This point is a common cause of misperception.

The family members should be encouraged to have positive regard for the individual. The individual may not be able to understand complex sentences. The family members should keep their communications simple and to the point. A simple "Hi," or "Bye," and "How are you doing?" can be very meaningful for the person.

The individual with schizophrenia and schizoaffective disorder can still perform certain chores around the house, and they should be allowed to volunteer for what they would like to do.

The sick family member may need assistance with keeping track of appointments and in getting to these appointments.

The family members should be educated about the symptoms and how they are amenable to medications. They should, therefore, encourage the individual to stay on their medications to ensure an optimal outcome.

The other family members should also be told to avoid loud open confrontation and criticism with the sick member and with each other. This type of behavior tends to increase the risk for relapse.

It is important that all members behave in a cordial and respectful manner with each other and with the sick family member.

Last but not least, educate others about the fact that schizophrenia is a real illness. It is not a weakness of the mind or a faintness of the heart.

Avoid a critical tone when interacting with the person and do not raise your voice. Do not try to induce guilt or claim that his or her illness is causing a family member to be ill in grief over their illness.

It is natural to feel anxious and sad about illness in any family member, but one should not give in to despair. It is important to remember and take heart from the fact that the situation can improve and that the illness is very treatable. A silver lining sometimes is that the family can be even stronger for having cared for a member that has an illness.

Be respectful and calm and try to be helpful in whatever way you can. Even small acts of generosity and kindness go a long way. Try to use simple words and do not use complicated phrases or very abstract ideas with individuals that suffer from schizophrenia or schizoaffective disorder. Their illness makes it difficult for them to decipher the meaning of proverbs and metaphorical language.

ARE SCHIZOPHRENIC AND SCHIZOAFFECTIVE DISORDER PATIENTS DANGEROUS?

Most such patients are not dangerous. Individuals with schizoaffective disorder may have a higher level of impulsivity. When treated, they are often helpful to others. Sensationalistic reporting of isolated cases of violence tends to give an exaggerated sense of the dangerousness associated with mental illness. When treated and stable, these individuals do not have a higher level of violence.

Each, however, is unique, and the risk level should be assessed on an individual basis.

ARE INDIVIDUALS WITH SCHIZOPHRENIA DISABLED?

Schizophrenia is an illness that can be quite disabling but does not always have to be. Social Security Disability payments may provide some financial support when the individual is not able to work or engage in meaningful employment to support him or herself.

Some individuals with schizophrenia can overcome their illness and do engage in meaningful employment. They can work effectively, have relationships, raise families, and make useful contributions to society just like many others without the illness.

CAN MEDICATIONS CURE SCHIZOPHRENIA?

It seems that early treatment with medications and supportive interventions can be curative in some cases. About 42% of individuals do not have a recurrence after their first episode is treated. It is important that the stress level of the individual in the first year of recovery is reduced as much as possible. Sometimes removal from a stressful setting can be very therapeutic.

The treatment of the first episode should last at least a year and then taper off, and discontinuation should be undertaken under the supervision of a psychiatrist. Medications should be reinstituted at the first signs of a relapse into prior symptoms.

For chronic symptoms, medications should be continued indefinitely as the risk of relapse is high without medications.

WHAT ARE SOME WAYS TO INCREASE COMPLIANCE?

Some ways to increase the regularity of taking medications by the patient, also known as medication compliance, are as follows:

1. Don't let the medication run out.

2. Have enough refills and fill them in time.

3. Apps offered by various pharmacies can offer reminders and automatically send a notice to the pharmacy for refills when it is time to refill medications.

4. Ask your psychiatrist to minimize the number of doses to once or twice a day.

5. Use a pill container that can keep all your medications for a certain time together. Some pill containers have built-in alarms that sound when it is time to take your medication.

6. Associate the taking of medications with a daily routine such as brushing your teeth etc.

7. If you miss a dose, just take the next dose at the scheduled time. Do not double up on the dose in such situations.

8. Consider getting on Depot antipsychotics such as Risperdal Consta, Haldol Dec., Prolixin Dec or Invega Sustenna that can be given every 2 to 4 weeks.

HOW CAN PATIENTS SUCCESSFULLY MANAGE THEIR SYMPTOMS RELATED TO SCHIZOPHRENIA OR SCHIZOAFFECTIVE DISORDER?

When the right dose and the right combination of medications are found, the symptoms can be reduced and even eliminated. This can help the person regain their life and relationships. They can resume an interest in their prior pursuits once the illness has stabilized.

Many individuals with schizophrenia learn to recognize their symptoms and are comfortable with the nature of the illness. They are not unduly distracted by their symptoms and can ignore hallucinations and focus on what they want to focus on.

Patients who successfully manage their illness stick to the doses that keep them stable, and avoid the use of alcohol or drugs. They have a limited number of supportive friends and family members they can count on. They have hobbies that they enjoy and also engage in activities that they find meaningful in their lives.

The right medication regimen can make all of the above possible.

WHY IS THERE A TEMPTATION TO STOP MEDICATION?

One of the key motivators for stopping medications is unmanaged side effects or worries about long-term side effects.

Most side effects can be managed or reduced, and a consultation with the prescribing doctor should remedy this problem.

Regarding the long-term side effects such as tardive dyskinesia; the risk can be reduced by monitoring for the emergence of involuntary movements. This is part of the protocol of treatment for schizophrenia in every treatment setting. If the movements are detected early, a change in dose or placement on clozapine can be considered.

The risk of tardive dyskinesia is significantly lower with the new generation antipsychotics.

For the side effect of metabolic syndrome, dietary interventions and exercise can help. A change of antipsychotic may also be considered if there is significant weight gain. If the elevation of cholesterol or triglycerides is significant, lipid lowering medications and antidiabetic medications such as metformin can also help in curtailing and reducing these side effects.

One of the more insidious reasons for noncompliance is the feeling of having made a full recovery. Although there is a significant rate of remission from the first episode, many individuals do require continuing treatment for schizophrenia.

Any plans for discontinuation of medications should, therefore, be made in collaboration with the treating doctor. He or she can monitor for the re-emergence of any symptoms.

The last but by no means insignificant reason is the stigma still attached to mental illness. The only way to decrease this is to provide information and education.

Despite the fact that there are many known and unknown causes of schizophrenia, at the end of the day, it is essentially a biological illness. It is similar in many ways to other biological illness such as hypertension, arthritis, or heart disease. It responds favorably to the right treatment.

If, for example, you do not feel stigmatized about hypertension, or your arthritis, you should similarly not feel stigmatized by having schizophrenia and needing to take medication for it. To not get treatment would be to invite suffering and there is no reason to suffer when treatment is so effective.

The temptation to stop medication can lead to a vicious circle. Once you start, it is hard to get out of the noncompliance cycle due to diminishing insight that comes with the reemergence of symptoms.

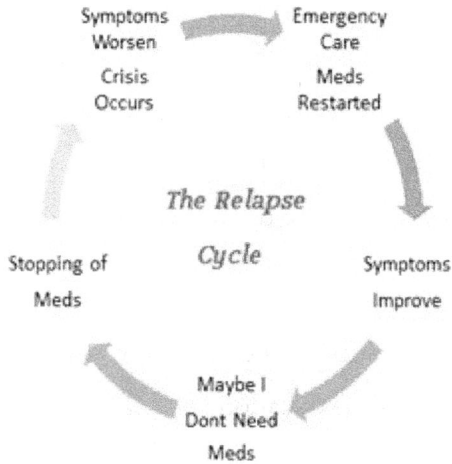

Symptoms
Worsen

Crisis
Occurs

Emergency
Care

Meds
Restarted

The Relapse

Cycle

Stopping of
Meds

Symptoms

Improve

Maybe I
Dont Need
Meds

The Key to Avoiding
Relapse is to
Stay On The Meds

HOW DOES INSIGHT DEVELOP OVER TIME?

In the acute phase of the illness of schizophrenia or schizoaffective disorder, the person is totally enveloped by his or her false beliefs and delusions. This lack of insight can be so dense that no rays of reality reach the waking consciousness. The person is truly in the dark.

Fortunately, the medications begin to work fast. There is often an improvement in even the first week of treatment with antipsychotic medications.

The first symptoms to improve are sleep and agitation due to the sedating effects of the medication. Then the hallucinations begin to decrease in a matter of days. With continuing treatment, the delusions begin to fade away day by day.

As improvement continues, the person begins to reflect in their quiet moments and starts to notice how their thinking in the past was perhaps a little strange. With continued treatment, they may realize that the beliefs were indeed "way out there." These insights are not usually proclaimed aloud. They do, however, reveal themselves by greater cooperation and compliance with treatment.

Many patients often achieve a total remission of their delusions and hallucinations. Other patients do not achieve total remission but still find significant relief. Their hallucinations are not as frequent or loud, and they can ignore them more easily. The delusions are also less troublesome due to the waning of their intensity. The person can tolerate an alternate reality other than that of their delusions. With continued treatment, the delusions grow fainter and do not cloud the judgment to the degree that they did before.

ARE UNUSUAL BELIEFS A SIGN OF MENTAL ILLNESS?

Unusual and bizarre beliefs held apart from the rest of the community that the person lives in can be a sign of mental illness. Sometimes, however, they are not a sign of mental illness, as explained below.

Some very bright and eccentric individuals march to their own drum and hold bizarre or unusual beliefs but are not necessarily mentally ill. Some famous scientists and artists may fit this profile. They do not suffer from hallucinations or delusions and have not lost touch with reality. They may, however, choose not to "heed reality" by a voluntary and competent choice.

Some individuals may have a personality disorder such as schizotypal personality disorder. Such individuals can hold unusual beliefs but do not suffer from hallucinations or delusions. Their contact with reality is intact.

Unusual beliefs may be shared by groups of people as in a cult. They are responding to indoctrination but otherwise have an intact reality testing system.

Large organized religions have beliefs that may be considered "illogical" by some other people. These unusual beliefs can be articles of faith and, some would argue, make some of these individuals more functional. Their belief in a loving higher power or deity can be considred unusual by atheists. But this belief can give them faith and hope in a time when their reality may be harsh and seemingly hopeless.

At such times, shared beliefs, even if seemingly illogical, are good for the person if they provide a reason to strive for a better day in the future. Religious articles of faith can inspire great acts of courage, sacrifice, and selfless service. Holding to such a belief, even if "illogical", cannot be considered a mental illness.

HOW DOES SCHIZOPHRENIA AFFECT FAMILY MEMBERS?

Family members may be saddened by the illness and be baffled by the symptoms that it produces. They should, however, not despair or blame themselves or the person with the illness for this. No one factor is responsible for the causation of schizophrenia.

It is important to keep a positive and optimistic attitude by recognizing that treatment is available. Sometimes, it takes more than one trial of medications to find the right combination. Most individuals diagnosed with schizophrenia can achieve a remission in their symptoms and lead productive and contented lives.

WHAT IS THE ROLE OF PARENTING IN THE CAUSATION OF SCHIZOPHRENIA?

Schizophrenia was at one time thought to be generated through the rearing of the child by cold and aloof parents who gave mixed and ambivalent signals about the acceptability and essential value of the child.

The parental approach was intellectualized, and emotional expressions were inhibited in such parents. The theory was called the theory of the schizophrenogenic mother, although fathers could also fit that stereotype.

There seems to be a kernel of truth in this theory even though the overall cause of schizophrenia seems to be much more complex.

Needless to say, if the parent is remote and barely emotionally "there" it does not help. A hypercritical or rejecting parent can also damage the basic sense of ego integrity in the growing child. If this is combined with a genetic vulnerability for the illness, the chances of the onset of schizophrenia may be increased.

The situation would be akin to that of a child who has a strong family history of diabetes who is assigned to a sedentary life without play and a diet rich in carbohydrates. The risk for developing diabetes in such a child would be higher compared to a child that has no family history of diabetes.

In an emotionally sterile and rejecting climate, an individual may be more vulnerable when he or she can find no anchor to define himself or herself. Such a frigid emotional climate may add to the splitting of the mind from emotions, a hallmark of schizophrenia.

Having said this, most parents are loving and may have raised the child perfectly in every way. An inopportune infection at a vulnerable period combined with other factors may be the main cause for the development of schizophrenia.

Most parents are blameless for the development of schizophrenia in their child. There is, however, some small validity in the idea of the schizophrenogenic parent.

WHAT IS A COMMUNITY MENTAL HEALTH CENTER?

A Community Mental Health Center is a subsidized mental health care center that offers free or prorated services according to a patient's ability to pay.

Most of these centers are run by the local county government. Sometimes the services may be contracted out to one or more private agencies.

Many well-run community mental health centers still exist across the country, and they do provide valuable services. You can find their local address and contact information by visiting the web page of your local county government or doing a search on one of the web search engines such as Yahoo or Google.

What is the prognosis when a person is treated with effective medications?

The prognosis is good.

Medications can help an individual take control of his or her life again. With the right medications, many of the symptoms of schizophrenia and schizoaffective disorder can be reduced significantly.

WHAT ARE THE SIGNS OF RELAPSE IN A PERSON WITH SCHIZOPHRENIA OR SCHIZOAFFECTIVE DISORDER?

Some of the signs of relapse may be as follows:

The person may exhibit a growing isolation from others.

They may neglect self-care and ADLs.

They may avoid activities that they used to enjoy.

They may become loud, boisterous and overly excitable and unusually happy.

Their activity level may be increased.

They may claim to hear a voice or voices.

They may be observed to be talking to themselves or an unseen entity.

They may express bizarre or paranoid ideas about conspiracies and plots to harm them.

They may sleep less than before.

They may engage in risky behavior such as speeding or drinking alcohol and using drugs.

They may engage in unusually promiscuous sexual behavior.

They may talk more than normal and in a louder volume.

They may seem unusually opinionated and unusually quick to snap at anybody over even minor disagreements.

If these symptoms and signs are observed, they should be referred to a psychiatrist for an adjustment of the medications.

Sometimes even a minor adjustment in the medications can make a big difference.

How can discontinuation of some medications help?

Sometimes discontinuation of certain meds may be what is needed.

For example, antidepressants and some antipsychotics with partial dopamine stimulant properties may need to be discontinued as they can precipitate manic and psychotic symptoms or make them worse.

SHOULD I TELL OTHERS ABOUT MY DIAGNOSIS?

It is important to let close family members know if you are diagnosed with schizophrenia so that they may offer support. They can also be your advocates when you go to the doctor. A family member or friend can also help collaborate your care with the different agencies.

You do not need to tell your coworkers or casual acquaintances if you are diagnosed with schizophrenia or schizoaffective disorder.

At work, some organizations are very supportive of individuals with disabilities. It is against the law to discriminate against those with disabilities in most countries. Enforcement of the law, however, varies.

Depending on your situation, you should discuss with your family and loved ones the matter of whether disclosure to your employee will work towards your best interests.

If the person with schizophrenia or schizoaffective disorder is stabilized and has no visible side effects, they cannot often be distinguished from those without the diagnosis.

WHAT KIND OF CHALLENGES DO FAMILIES AND FRIENDS ENCOUNTER?

In the beginning, it can be difficult to understand the nature of the illness and some of the symptoms can be frightening and intimidating.

Sometimes, the risk of aggression is higher and sometimes it does not exist. If there is any risk of physical harm to any family member due to aggression generated by a delusion or manic state, due precautions should be taken, and the patient must be taken to the hospital for stabilization of the acute state.

Education is the key to warding off anxiety. Although close friends and family are at a higher risk of violence from the individual in the acute phase of schizophrenic or schizoaffective disorder illness, for the most part, the individual with these illnesses is not violent.

Due precautions should be taken, however, if there have been past threats, a history of violence or growing agitation.

WHAT ARE SOME SOURCES OF SUPPORT IN THE COMMUNITY?

The following additional resources may exist in your community:

1. Residential day program

2. Skilled nursing facilities that house individuals with schizophrenia and schizoaffective disorder

3. The local church and pastor

4. Local churches, synagogues, mosques and temples may also be a resource. The clergy attending these places of worship may be educated about mental illness and can sometimes be a resource. Some of the major religions have a compassionate view of mental illness and may have free clinics where treatment and support can be obtained.

5. NAMI or the National Association for Mental Illness has been mentioned and is a great resource for families and patients. Local support groups can be found at their website. You can search by typing in NAMI on a search engine such as Google.

6. Homeless shelters and soup kitchens can be a source of support for those in acute need of shelter or food.

WHAT CAN AN INDIVIDUAL WITH SCHIZOPHRENIA DO TO GET ALONG BETTER WITH OTHERS?

The ability to get along with others can be improved by the teaching of social skills. Some of the skills listed below can be practiced with family or friends to improve the patient's ability to get along with others. It can allow for better experiences with the public and an enhanced quality of life. Some of these skills are elementary but should not be taken for granted. Some training in even the basic social skills such as the ones mentioned below can make a world of difference.

Some points worth training for are as follows:

1. Say, "Hello," when you meet a person.

2. Say, "Goodbye," when you leave.

3. When you meet a person, to start the conversation, ask, "How are You?" or "How is your day going so far?"

4. When you need something, ask rather than tell. For example, say, "Could you do this for me?" instead of, "Do this for me right now."

5. Say, "Please," when requesting something.

6. Say, "Thank you," when your request is granted.

7. Make eye contact but do not glare.

8. If you like something about a place or person, provide a compliment. You can say something like. "You do a great job in getting me to my appointment/getting me on the right medication," etc. Pay a compliment if you receive good service or if something pleases you.

9. Learn small talk such as asking an opinion about recent news, the "the game" or the "the weather" etc.

10. Learn grooming skills.

11. Maintain good hygiene.

12. Learn how to refuse offers of alcohol or drugs,

    e.g. "It interacts with my meds," *because it does.*

13. Practice being relaxed around others. Take a deep breath or two if you are feeling anxious, relax your muscles and imagine something pleasant to help you feel relaxed. When you are tense or jittery, it increases everyone else's anxiety since many are already anxious about your diagnosis and what it means. Many people don't understand that not all individuals with mental illnesses are violent. Your ability to stay relaxed will help dispel this myth.

WHY ARE SHELTERS IMPORTANT?

A shelter of some kind can be all important in places that experience temperature extremes. The risk from extreme temperatures is further increased with the antipsychotic medications that are prescribed to individuals with schizophrenia and schizoaffective disorder. Exposure to temperatures above 90 degrees Fahrenheit can increase the risk for heat stroke and heat exhaustion. This is because the anticholinergic effects of antipsychotics such as thorazine and medications given to prevent side effects such as Cogentin can decrease sweating and the ability to regulate temperature.

In the winter, there seems to be a higher vulnerability to cold and hypothermia as some antipsychotics dilate blood vessels and may increase heat loss in cold weather. Inappropriate attire can be a symptom of schizophrenia, hence it is doubly important for the individual to dress appropriately for the weather.

HOW CAN A DEDICATED CASE MANAGER HELP A PERSON WITH SCHIZOPHRENIA?

A dedicated case manager can make a world of difference for the individual who suffers from schizophrenia. He or she can:

- Help in arranging for transportation to groups, meetings, appointments

- Monitor your progress

- Help you with applying for benefits

How a Case Manager Can Help You		
Arranges transportation to groups, meetings, appointments	Monitors Your Progress	Helps you to apply for benefits

HOW SHOULD AN INDIVIDUAL WITH SCHIZOPHRENIA BEHAVE WHEN INTERACTING WITH THE POLICE?

When you are asked by the police to do something, do it and be respectful while doing so. Do it even if it does not make sense to you.

Let them know you are not armed.

Display your hands where they can be seen.

Do not keep your hands in your pocket.

If your face is covered by a hoodie, uncover it.

Do not make any threatening statements.

Do not issue any threats towards the officer or anyone else.

Remember, the police are your friends. You are safest when you are with them. Many of them have some training on mental health issues and will be sympathetic.

The police do carry lethal force weapons in the United States. They are human beings just like everyone else and must contend with dangerous situations day in and day out. If they feel threatened, they are trained to respond to the threat at whatever level is needed.

If you make threatening statements or keep your hands in your pocket, they do not know that you are not carrying a gun.

If you do not cooperate but make threatening moves, there is a very real chance that you could get shot or killed.

The police do not want to do this. They want to help and are there to serve and protect. At the end of the day, they want to go home to their families. They have a difficult job and deserve a lot of respect.

Make it easy for yourself and them by being cooperative with them. Listen to them, be respectful and follow their directions. This will ensure your safety and will also ensure further care for you.

WHAT ARE SOME PSYCHOSOCIAL CHALLENGES ASSOCIATED WITH MENTAL ILLNESS?

There are many psychosocial hurdles for patients with schizophrenia and other major mental illness. Some of these are listed below.

- Unmet financial needs, poverty

- Poor housing

- Poor nutrition

- Unemployment

- Underemployment

- Undertreatment of medical issues

- Disrupted relationships

- Need of training about coping skills

- Need for anger management skill training

- Treatment of alcohol and substance abuse problems

- High rates of incarceration

- Underfunding of public mental health programs

WHAT CAN THE FAMILY DO TO BE HELPFUL?

The family members should take a shared responsibility for helping their loved one. The task can be overwhelming for one person alone. They can help in some of the following ways:

- Encourage the patient to take their medications daily.

- Encourage the patient to keep their appointments.

- Be supportive.

- Be willing to listen to any problems.

- Help with any complicated directions or instructions or ask the doctor to explain these if there is a lack of clarity.

- Provide structure and routine for the person. Having set times for meal times and other activities decreases ambivalence in the surroundings and this is useful.

- Share responsibility with other family members and seek support for yourself if you feel emotionally exhausted.

WHAT IS THE DIFFERENCE BETWEEN GROUP THERAPY AND A SUPPORT GROUP?

Group therapy is a form of therapy wherein individuals suffering from a similar condition meet on a regular basis to discuss their problems and get support and guidance from each other <u>and the therapist</u>. There is usually a fee or charge for attending the group, and regular attendance is required.

A support group is a form of therapy where individuals gather on a regular basis to discuss their common issues and offer support and encouragement to each other. A therapist is not required for a support group. More mature members of the group can take on leadership roles and be mentors and guides for those who are in the initial stages of their recovery. It is a great tool and it is free. Attendance in a support group is voluntary but regular attendance is encouraged.

The support group can be helpful when the patient has stabilized to some extent in their recovery.

The National Alliance for the Mentally Ill (NAMI) offers a listing of local support groups on their webpage.

The NAMI website is at

<u>http://www.nami.org/</u>

If you click on the Find Support tab on this website, you can access support groups in your area.

They also have an 800 help line at 1800-950-6264 or 1800-950-NAMI. The help line is open from 10 am to 6 pm Eastern Standard Time.

NAMI is a great organization that advocates for the rights of the mentally ill at the highest level of government.

Similar organizations exist in other countries.

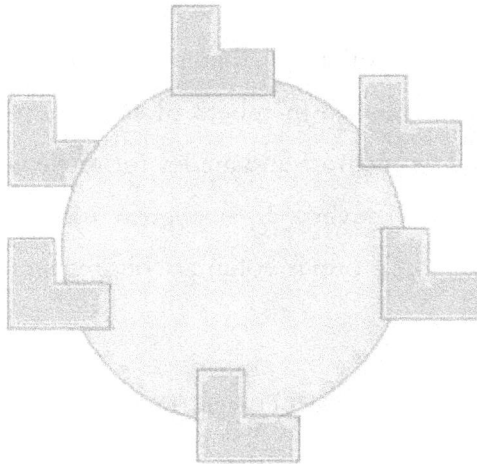

**Support Groups can be very helpful when available.
Support Groups are not led by a therapist**

Group Therapy is a type of therapy led by a trained clinician. It can be very helpful as well.

HOW CAN A PERSON WITH SCHIZOPHRENIA GET HELP IN CASE OF AN ACUTE CRISIS?

- The person with schizophrenia may walk into the emergency room and ask for help.

- He or she may also call 911 and get transportation to the local emergency room, especially if he or she is having thoughts of harming self or others.

- If the person with acute mental illness is exhibiting dangerous behaviors, anyone can call for police assistance. The police have the power and authority to transport the person under a mental health law active in most places around the world. In the United States, it is called a 72-hour hold or a 5150. The purpose of this is to secure the safety of the person afflicted with mental illness and also secure the safety of others. It also allows for mental health professionals to evaluate the condition of the patient and make a further determination about immediate and long-term mental health needs of the individual.

- If inpatient course of treatment is recommended and the patient refuses, a continuation can be filed or what is called a 5250. This petition must be heard by an officer of the court to verify the facts of the case and to ascertain whether circumstances justify the case for involuntary hospitalization. It is ultimately in the hands of the court to make a determination of what is needed in the best interests of the individual.

- From a legal perspective, the issue for the court is the balance of the civil rights of the individual vs. the greater risk of harm to the person and public from the unrestrained movement of the seriously mentally ill person in his untreated state.

- It is important for the patient to remember that everyone is trying to help them. They should try to be cooperative, despite the mistrust and fear that they may feel. By being cooperative, you will receive the help you need more efficiently and will start feeling better in a few days.

- Do not be afraid of trying medications for the voices and fears. Ask the doctor to prescribe medications to prevent any side effects. Remember to thank the doctors and nurses who are trying to help you. Ask questions if you have any.

HOW DIFFICULT IS IT TO GET AN APPOINTMENT AT A LOCAL COMMUNITY MENTAL HEALTH CENTER?

It can be as easy as looking up the number in the phone book or on the internet. On Google, one can type in, "Community Mental Health Center," or "Mental Health Center," and the search engine will automatically bring up the local mental health center. One can also be more specific in the location of the mental health center.

For example, if I type in, "Fresno County Mental Health Center telephone," it brings up the following page. One of the items gives the number for mental health.

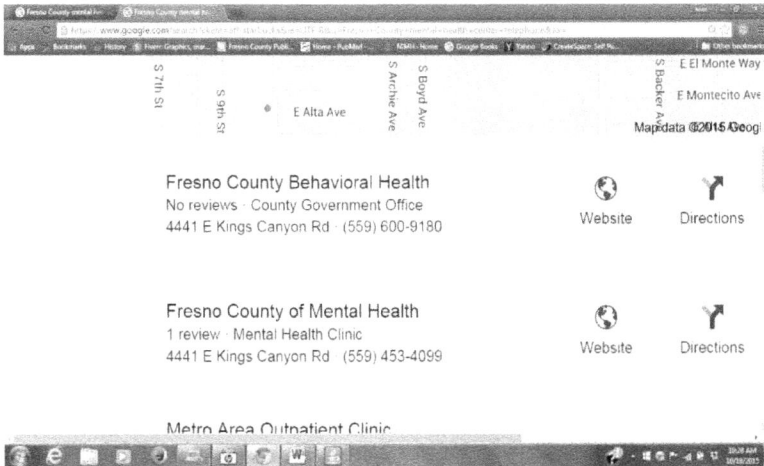

Instead of mental health, sometimes the word behavioral health may be used. If I call any of these numbers, I can get further guidance on how to access services. The staff is trained to be friendly and helpful.

UPON RELEASE FROM A PRISON OR JAIL, WHAT RESOURCES ARE AVAILABLE FOR THE TREATMENT OF MENTAL ILLNESS?

- If you suffer from mental illness and the symptoms are severe and not controlled, you may be sent to a state hospital for further stabilization.

- If an individual is stable, they are given a month's supply of medications and an appointment with the local mental health center.

- The prisons have case managers that coordinate care in the community upon release. If the individual is on parole, parole clinics are available.

- Compliance with treatment is often a condition of the parole. It is important, therefore, to keep these appointments because not maintaining your treatments may lead to your return to jail or prison.

IS HELP AVAILABLE AT COLLEGES FOR MENTAL HEALTH NEEDS?

Yes, many colleges and universities do have mental health clinics where counseling and medication treatment can be provided. The regents and administrators of the university, if they are wise and farsighted, will recognize the following facts:

Young adulthood at a college can be a stressful time when the person is dealing with

1. Separation from family and friends

2. The burden of new academic tasks

3. Incurring of significant loans to pay for the education

4. Early twenties is the time for the onset of many of the serious mental illnesses such as schizophrenia, bipolar disorder, and depression

5. A sense of identity that is undergoing a shift into their future adult role. Compromises have to be made because one realizes that one cannot be all of the things one imagined possible in their idealistic youth

Given the fact that many of the serious illnesses such as schizophrenia have their onset in the twenties when most individuals are at college, it is all the more important that such help is made available. Early recognition and treatment can be lifesaving as the person is often away from family and may not have much in the way of local support and resources.

In a faceless crowd of newcomers to a university, it is easy for the person with an evolving illness to go unrecognized and fail to get help in a timely manner.

HOW CAN THE FAMILY MEDICAL LEAVE ACT BE HELPFUL?

The family medical leave act, FMLA, was instituted in the United States in 1993 with the help of President Bill Clinton. It is a federal law requiring that employers provide to employees job-protected unpaid leave for qualified medical and family reasons. Some employers may even provide a period of paid leave to deal with the illness.

Many other countries provide similar leave plans.

This leave can be used to help a family member or to deal with a personal illness that requires a lengthy period of recovery and recuperation. The advantage of the law is that you cannot be fired from your job for using such leave.

For someone dealing with the illness of schizophrenia in a family member, such leave can be a good thing to have available. Some individuals may need to continue working as they cannot afford to take unpaid leave. In such cases, other sources of support may be available. A case worker can offer further guidance in this regard.

CHAPTER 4

TREATMENT CONSIDERATIONS

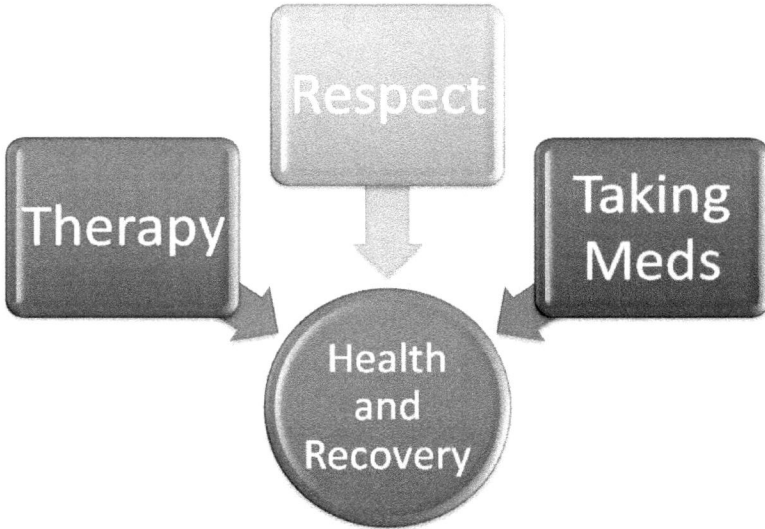

WHAT IS A TREATMENT TEAM IN A MENTAL HEALTH SETTING?

A Treatment Team is a group of professionals from different helping professions who work together in collaboration to help the individual with mental illness.

It has been shown in multiple studies that a combined treatment team approach is better than only using medications or only using psychotherapy. The best results are obtained by using multiple modes, à la the bio-psycho-social modes, to meet the diverse needs of the individual.

The patient should also be included in the treatment team. He or she can play an important role in deciding the treatment goals. Compliance is also likely to be higher when the patient is actively involved in the formulation of a treatment goal.

A TEAM APPROACH TO
TREATMENT IS ALWAYS BETTER

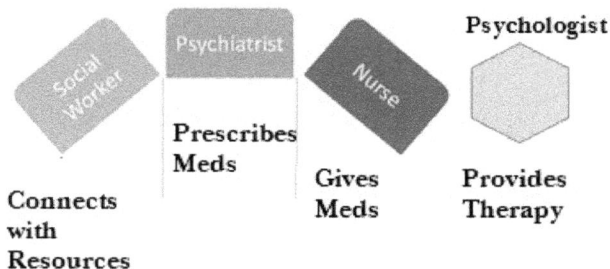

Social Worker

Psychiatrist

Nurse

Psychologist

Prescribes Meds

Gives Meds

Provides Therapy

Connects with Resources

The treatment team is usually comprised of the following professionals:

- Psychiatrist

- Psychologist

- Social Worker

- Case Worker

- Rec Therapist

- Nursing Staff

- Primary Care Provider as needed

- Correctional counselor if patient is in prison

- Family member or clergy if requested by the patient

- Each patient is also assigned a case manager who helps coordinate implementation of the treatment plan

The case manager may be the social worker or another designated member of staff. It is important for there to be a primary contact person who helps the patient navigate the maze that a healthcare system can be.

It is important for the team to be patient-centered. This means that the patient should be allowed to participate in the formulation of the treatment goals for his or her care. Defined goals should be set that are reasonable, and concrete steps should be delineated that can be taken to help realize that goal. The goals should also have some defined measurable quality.

It is important that any alcohol and substance abuse issues are addressed.

It is also important that any medical needs of the patient are addressed promptly. Follow-up of chronic medical issues should be arranged. The patient should be educated about the importance of compliance with psychiatric and medical treatments and medications.

HOW CAN A PERSON WITH SCHIZOPHRENIA BECOME MORE ORGANIZED?

Schizophrenia may affect attention and working memory to a minor degree. This effect is understandably greater when the symptoms are acute and uncontrolled.

Once the acute symptoms are controlled, some minor organizational strategies can help the person stay organized.

Some patients find that keeping a diary with a calendar is helpful in jotting down important dates of appointments. It can also be helpful for noting ideas and important information about medications, telephone numbers, and directions.

Generally speaking, simpler methods of keeping organized are better than high tech methods. The high-tech devices and apps can sometimes generate more confusion and distraction.

Also, some patients with schizophrenia may be wary of using technological gadgets.

If they do not have such issues, however, and are fairly adept at using a smartphone or other devices, they can be allowed to use such devices for keeping their information organized.

Another way to help the patient stay organized and healthy is to provide pill boxes that contain compartments for their morning and/or evening meds, as the case may be.

The medication regimens should be simplified whenever possible to once a day or at the most twice a day administration whenever possible.

Depot antipsychotics may be administered once every 2 to 4 weeks. This use of depot antipsychotics greatly increases compliance and decreases relapse rates across the board.

Use of to-do lists or checklists should be encouraged. These lists should not become too lengthy or cumbersome or they will not be looked at and will not be acted upon. There is something inherently unpleasant about a long to-do list.

WHAT IS A RELAPSE CYCLE?

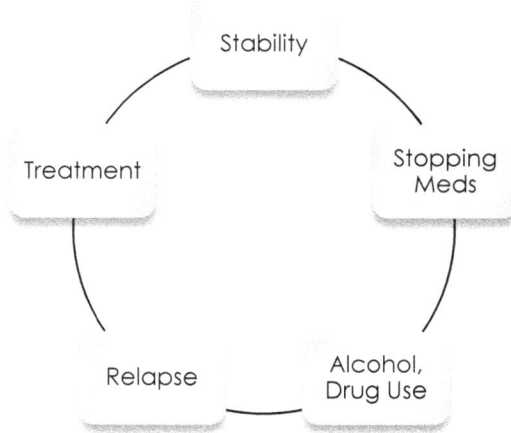

Stability

Stopping
Meds

Treatment

Relapse

Alcohol,
Drug Use

A relapse cycle is a repeating pattern in which the person stops taking their medication when they start feeling better. This often leads to a relapse of the illness until help is obtained to restart the recovery cycle. The person may discontinue meds again and the process goes through the same steps again. This is called the relapse cycle. Each relapse is full of hazards, and the results can be harmful to the individual and others. Drugs and substance abuse are often contributing factors to the relapse cycle. One should follow the simple rule below to avoid the relapse cycle.

WHAT ARE THE MOST IMPORTANT LESSONS FOR PREVENTING THE RELAPSE CYCLE?

These lessons are as follows:

- Continue your medication even when you are feeling better.

- Medications for schizophrenia are like medications for blood pressure; they need to be taken for the long term.

- Say, "No," to Alcohol and Drugs every time the opportunity comes up. They are known to directly cause psychosis and worsen the underlying psychosis that is being treated.

What is the History of Treating Schizophrenia?

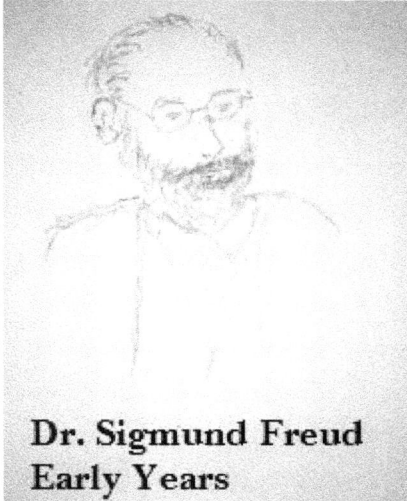

**Dr. Sigmund Freud
Early Years**

In the early 20th century, Sigmund Freud (1856-1939) became a major influence as he explored psychodynamic factors that contributed to different states of anxiety, depression and thought disturbance. His insights were remarkable but did not always translate well into the treatment of those with schizophrenia and schizoaffective disorder.

Other therapies were also tried including prolonged sleep therapy, fever therapy, insulin coma therapy and induction of seizures by chemicals or with electricity. Many of these treatments had unpredictable outcomes and side effects.

Egas Moniz, a neurologist, became famous for frontal lobotomies to treat agitation in individuals with psychotic agitation. In 1949, the Nobel Prize in Physiology or Medicine was awarded to him "for his discovery of the therapeutic value of leucotomy in certain psychoses."

He shared this prize with Walter Rudolf Hess, who did some brilliant research on the functional organization of the brain. The lobotomy procedure gained notoriety for being overused in an era when no effective treatment was available for the treatment of violent agitation found in some individuals with psychosis. The procedure is no longer used with the arrival of effective medications.

The 1950s were a landmark decade in the history of psychiatry. This was the decade in which an effective medication was discovered for the first time with the advent of chlorpromazine, a medication originally designed for other purposes.

The effectiveness of chlorpromazine was a chance discovery that only became widely recognized after the publication of a seminal paper by a team of French psychiatrists comprising Pierre Deniker, Jean Delay and JM Harl in 1952. They reported a remarkable calming effect of this agent in agitated psychotic patients that went beyond mere sedation. It actually lessened the hallucinations and eased the intensity of delusions.

Soon, chlorpromazine became widely prescribed by doctors in psychiatric hospitals across the world. Others also noted that there was a remarkable improvement of symptoms for the first time in many individuals who had suffered from tormenting hallucinations and fears for years. It seemed almost like a miracle to some. The possibility of a better life through chemistry had indeed arrived, or so it seemed.

There was much excitement and optimism among doctors, administrators and politicians. For the first time, doctors had an agent that could decrease the voices and ease the fears that had plagued individuals with schizophrenia.

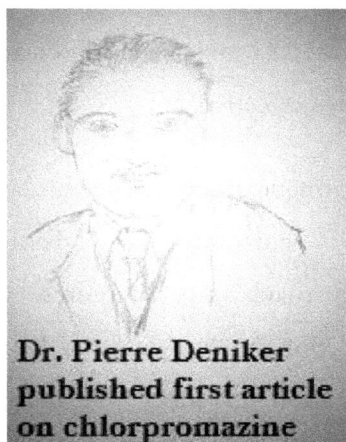

Dr. Pierre Deniker published first article on chlorpromazine

In the flush of this optimism, plans were made to close down the large state hospitals and to only seek community-based treatment for those with serious mental illness. This mass group think did not realize that the medications were not always 100 percent effective and that these patients still needed social support to make it on their own.

The state hospitals, in fact, did empty their wards, and many were discharged to the streets. The hope was that the patients could follow up at the mental health centers in the community.

It was only later that we learned how many of these individuals with chronic mental illness were ending up in our jails and prisons. This was, in part, due to poor planning and the absence of adequate support structures for those discharged from long-term institutions.

The drift of the mentally ill into our jails and prisons has underscored the point that pharmacological treatment is only one aspect of treatment. Medications are not a cure-all, neither are they a panacea that is always effective.

Furthermore, the treatment of a pervasive and global illness such as schizophrenia or schizoaffective disorder requires a multidisciplinary approach. It requires that psychiatrists, psychologists, social workers, nursing and other disciplines work together in collaboration to meet the different needs of the individual. Only such a collaboration can ensure an optimum level of care for the individual.

The advent of chlorpromazine was followed by other antipsychotics such as haloperidol, fluphenazine, trifluoperazine, perphenazine and thiothixene. None of these agents were more effective than the others and only differed in the type of side effects they were associated with. Later, clozapine was introduced. It truly had a greater level of efficacy but was also associated with a dangerous side effect of agranulocytosis in 1% of individuals who took it.

Agranulocytosis is the shutting down of the bone marrow that produces white blood cells amongst other things. The white blood cells are required to fight off infections. If their number falls below 3500, the risk for infections is increased. If there is a severe shutdown of WBC (white blood cell) production, the person can develop life-threatening infections.

The use of clozapine (Clozaril) therefore requires that the white blood cell count is monitored on a regular basis.

WHEN WERE THE NEW ANTIPSYCHOTICS INTRODUCED AND HOW ARE THEY DIFFERENT?

In the 1990s, a new generation of antipsychotic medications was introduced starting with risperidone. These were called the second generation antipsychotics or atypical antipsychotics. They were atypical because they did not have the "typical" side effects of the earlier class of antipsychotics such as tremors, acute muscle stiffness or tardive dyskinesia. Their arrival was greeted with great fanfare because they were found not to have the problematic parkinsonian side effects to the degree that the earlier antipsychotics had.

Clozapine was the first of the atypical antipsychotics but was not allowed in the United States till much later. The first atypical antipsychotic available for widespread use was risperidone, which came out in 1994.

Risperidone was followed by olanzapine, quetiapine, ziprasidone, aripiprazole, lurasidone and asenapine.

Clozapine is the most effective antipsychotic amongst all antipsychotics. Risperidone, olanzapine, and quetiapine seem to be more effective than the other atypical antipsychotics.

Clozapine, Olanzapine, and Risperidone, however, are more commonly implicated with a side effect called the metabolic syndrome. This syndrome is marked by weight gain, increased cholesterol and insulin resistance resulting in elevated blood sugars. The other atypical antipsychotic agents also carry a warning for the same side effect of metabolic syndrome but the risk of the metabolic syndrome appears to be less with them.

So the conundrum is that the effective antipsychotics have side effects, and those with fewer side effects are not always as effective.

Some individuals do seem to benefit from these medications that have fewer side effects. It is worth offering the more benign second generation antipsychotics to those for whom they are effective while monitoring for objective signs of improvement.

WHY IS IT IMPORTANT TO TREAT SYMPTOMS SOONER RATHER THAN LATER?

1. Early treatment of symptoms lessens suffering.

2. It also improves the long-term outlook.

3. The person whose schizophrenic illness is treated early is more likely to have a milder form of the illness in the long run.

4. There is a better chance for the continued and sustained remission of symptoms after the first year when treatment is provided early.

WHAT ARE THE CHALLENGES OF WORKING WITH SOMEONE EXPERIENCING SYMPTOMS OF PSYCHOSIS?

From a clinical perspective, working with a patient in the throes of a psychotic illness is one of the most challenging jobs any human being can have. There is an inherent distrust of the psychiatrist or other clinician who is trying to help. In some settings, there is a very real danger of being assaulted by an angry patient who is struggling with paranoia and a sense of persecution. Many clinicians working in the mental health field have been attacked by angry patients.

The clinician may be object of ire and anger for suggesting that the person needs treatment. The sickest patients sometimes need involuntary treatment. Initiating medications on a person who thinks they do not need them is always a high risk situation.

This is not universal, however, and some patients do retain insight of their illness. They find relief in knowing their condition has a name and are grateful for being provided the help that they need. They may later apologize for any outbursts that they may have had.

WHAT IS THE MOST CRUCIAL COMPONENT OF TREATING SCHIZOPHRENIA?

The mainstay treatment of schizophrenia and schizoaffective disorder is the proficient use of antipsychotic medications by a trained psychiatrist.

There are many medications now available that can help to diminish and sometimes eliminate the main symptoms such as hearing of voices, paranoia, and delusions.

In addition to medications, it is important that psychological and social interventions be also considered. They have an important therapeutic role in the treatment of these illnesses.

Below is illustrated the biopsychosocial model of treatment that encompasses different approaches to the treatment of schizophrenia and schizoaffective disorder.

WHAT IS THE BIOPSYCHOSOCIAL MODEL
OF TREATMENT?

This model of illness believes that most illnesses have a complex variety of contributing factors. These factors can be biological, social, or psychological. The treatment has to therefore address all three spheres.

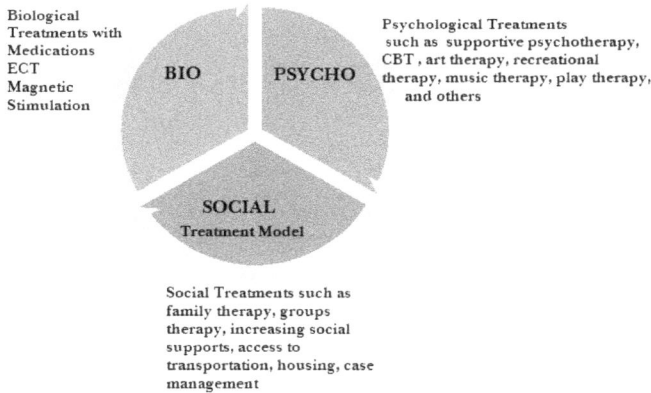

Biological Treatments with Medications ECT Magnetic Stimulation

BIO

PSYCHO

Psychological Treatments such as supportive psychotherapy, CBT, art therapy, recreational therapy, music therapy, play therapy, and others

SOCIAL
Treatment Model

Social Treatments such as family therapy, groups therapy, increasing social supports, access to transportation, housing, case management

WHAT KINDS OF MEDICATIONS ARE USED FOR TREATMENT?

Medications are used for two different symptom sets. These are the psychotic symptoms and mood symptoms that may accompany a psychotic illness.

These are depicted below.

Medications for Schizophrenia and Schizoaffective Disorder

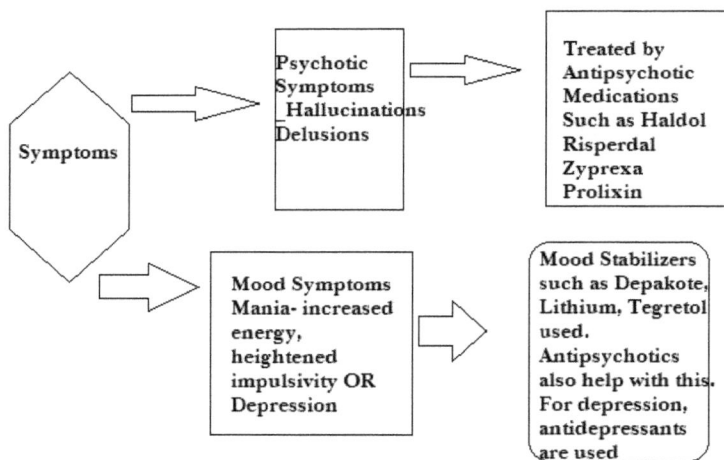

```
                          ┌──────────────┐              ┌──────────────────┐
                          │ Psychotic    │              │ Treated by       │
                          │ Symptoms     │   ═══════▷   │ Antipsychotic    │
           ═══════▷       │  Hallucina-  │              │ Medications      │
  ╱──────╲                │  tions       │              │ Such as Haldol   │
 │        │               │ Delusions    │              │ Risperdal        │
 │Symptoms│               │              │              │ Zyprexa          │
 │        │               └──────────────┘              │ Prolixin         │
  ╲──────╱                                              └──────────────────┘
           ═══════▷       ┌──────────────┐              ┌──────────────────┐
                          │ Mood Symptoms│              │ Mood Stabilizers │
                          │ Mania- in-   │   ═══════▷   │ such as Depakote,│
                          │ creased      │              │ Lithium, Tegretol│
                          │ energy,      │              │ used.            │
                          │ heightened   │              │ Antipsychotics   │
                          │ impulsivity  │              │ also help with   │
                          │ OR           │              │ this.            │
                          │ Depression   │              │ For depression,  │
                          └──────────────┘              │ antidepressants  │
                                                        │ are used         │
                                                        └──────────────────┘
```

HOW ARE ANTIPSYCHOTIC MEDICATIONS CLASSIFIED?

They are broadly classified into two groups

- The older or the first generation

- The newer or the second generation

WHAT ARE SOME FIRST GENERATION ANTIPSYCHOTICS?

Some of the first generation antipsychotic agents are listed below.

Haloperidol (Haldol): It is an effective antipsychotic that has minimal sedation effects or any side effects related to dizziness. The target dose is 10 to 20 mg. Sometimes lower doses are effective. It is available in a long-acting form as Haldol Decanoate that can be administered once a month.

Fluphenazine (Prolixin): It is another effective antipsychotic that has mild sedation effects. The side effects related to dizziness are minimal. The target dose is 10 to 20 mg. Sometimes lower doses are effective. It is available in a long-acting form, Prolixin Decanoate, that can be administered once every two to three weeks.

Trifluoperazine (Stelazine): Is less potent than Haldol or Prolixin but is more potent than Navane. It is effective in the dose range of 5 to 20 mg for most individuals. May need anticholinergic medications to prevent extra pyramidal side effects.

Thiothixene (Navane): Target dose of 10 to 30 mg or higher is effective. It has more sedating side effects.

Perphenazine (Trilafon): Target dose is 16 to 48 mg. It is sedating and may have some side effects of dizziness at higher doses.

Molindone (Moban): It is more sedating, has more risk for dizziness with rapid dose escalation. It is effective as an antipsychotic.

Loxapine (Loxitane): It is also sedating. It has more sedation, more risk for causing dizziness with rapid dose escalation. It is effective as an antipsychotic just like all the others. A few psychiatrists feel that it may be more effective in some cases due to its unique molecular structure that is chemically related to clozapine.

Chlorpromazine (Thorazine): It was the first antipsychotic to be introduced in 1952 and is still used effectively today. It is very sedating and is used for calming agitated patients and for insomnia in individuals with psychosis. It can cause dry mouth and constipation. The risk of dizziness exists if the dose is raised rapidly.

***

The first generation or older antipsychotics are particularly helpful for the positive symptoms such as hallucinations and delusions.

They also have the advantage of <u>not causing</u> the metabolic syndrome that is marked by weight gain and risk for elevated cholesterol and diabetes. However, they do have a higher incidence of side effects such as tremor, akathisia, and tardive dyskinesia.

In addition to the significant benefit for hallucinations and delusions, they do provide some degree of benefit for the negative symptoms as well.

This benefit may be masked, however, by the extrapyramidal side effects that produce symptoms similar to Parkinson's disease.

WHAT ARE THE SOME EFFECTIVE SECOND GENERATION ANTIPSYCHOTICS?

Some effective second generation antipsychotic agents are as follows:

- clozapine (Clozaril)

- risperidone (Risperdal)

- olanzapine (Zyprexa)

- quetiapine (Seroquel)

There some other atypical antipsychotics but they tend to vary in their effectiveness or are sometimes ineffective.

Amongst the atypical antipsychotics, clozapine is more efficacious than all other antipsychotics. It does, however, have some serious side effects in a few patients and is held in reserve for the cases that are refractory to other antipsychotics.

Some more details are as follows:

Clozapine (Clozaril/Fazaclo): This is a second generation antipsychotic used for those with treatment refractory schizophrenia or schizoaffective disorder. Weekly blood draws are required for the first six months to rule out a drop in white blood cells.

It can have remarkable benefits for some individuals and it works for both positive and negative symptoms of schizophrenia to a greater degree than any other antipsychotic. The target dose is 400 to 600 mg but sometimes lower doses are effective when used in conjunction with other antipsychotics. At higher doses, there is an increasing risk of side effects related to seizures, low white blood cell counts, constipation and other side effects.

One of the serious side effects associated with clozapine is a 1 percent risk of agranulocytosis (shutting down of the bone marrow that produces white blood cells to fight infections).

If agranulocytosis occurs, the clozapine needs to be stopped right away, and the person needs to be protected from opportunistic infection due to the lowered immunity. With the discontinuation of clozapine, the bone marrow usually recovers its function without complications. If the white count gets suppressed, the frequency of monitoring of the white blood cells is usually increased to twice a week until the white blood cell count bounces back to normal levels.

Olanzapine (Zyprexa): This is a second-generation antipsychotic. It is generally well tolerated with high compliance rates. The incidence of motor side effects such as acute muscle stiffness or tremor is low. It has a mild sedating effect that is higher at the higher doses. The usual starting dose is 10 to 15 mg with a target dose range of 15 to 30 mg. Sometimes doses up to 40 mg or higher are needed. The official upper dose is 20 mg, but higher doses are often required and are well tolerated.

Side effects related to olanzapine are weight gain, elevation of cholesterol and resistance to insulin in some patients, leading to elevation of blood sugar and diabetes mellitus. It is important to monitor body weight. If there is a rapid weight gain, consideration should be given to trying an alternative antipsychotic.

Quetiapine (Seroquel): This is an atypical antipsychotic with sedating qualities and with risk for causing dizziness. It is therefore started at a low dose and gradually titrated up. It may take a while for antipsychotic response and higher doses than the upper limit of 800 mg are sometimes needed to achieve a therapeutic response. It tends to have a lower risk for causing weight gain, or side effects related to tremor or acute muscle stiffness.

Risperidone (Risperdal): This is a second-generation antipsychotic that was one of the first of this class of second-generation antipsychotics. It is very effective for the control of positive symptoms of serious schizophrenic illness such as auditory hallucinations and delusions. The target dose is 4 to 6 mg, but sometimes higher doses are needed. When the acute symptoms have been stabilized, a lower dose may be able to maintain stability. The side effects related to tremor or muscle stiffness are also not prominent at doses less than 6 mgs. If these occur, benztropine (Cogentin) 1 mg two to three times a day offers relief from these side effects.

It is available as a long-acting intramuscular injection called Risperdal Consta. It is administered every two weeks.

Invega is a breakdown product of risperidone. It is offered as a tablet and a long-acting injection, Invega Sustenna, that is administered every four weeks.

WHAT ARE EXTRAPYRAMIDAL (EPS) SIDE EFFECTS AND PARKINSONIAN SIDE EFFECTS?

EPS side effects and parkinsonian side effects are the same thing. They are symptoms exhibited in Parkinson's disease and side effects when the parkinsonian syndrome is produced by antipsychotic medications.

These symptoms or side effects are as follows:

1. A resting tremor of the hand that can cause the hand to look as if it is rolling something. It is for this reason also called the "pill rolling" tremor.

2. Bradykinesia (Brady means slow, Kinesis is movement). This when muscle movements are slowed due to increased muscle tone.

3. Increased muscle tone and rigidity of movement. When muscles are moved, the muscles move in a cog wheeling manner.

4. Mask like face with decreased emotional expression due to bradykinesia related to the facial muscles.

5. Shuffling Gait.

6. Dystonia. This is an acute muscle contraction of a group of muscles.

Treatment: These symptoms and side effects can be easily treated and prevented by the addition of anticholinergic medications such as Cogentin, Artane, or Benadryl.

ARE EPS SIDE EFFECTS MORE LIKELY IN SOME POPULATIONS?

The EPS side effects described above may occur at higher rates in young people, and those of oriental descent.

As mentioned, they are easily prevented by using some of the medications mentioned earlier such as benztropine (Cogentin), trihexyphenidyl (Artane) or diphenhydramine (Benadryl) in low doses two to three times a day.

The acute muscle stiffness or dystonia is somewhat uncomfortable but not dangerous. It can be easily treated by an intramuscular injection of Benadryl 50 mgs or Cogentin 2 mg. Thereafter, the patient should be prescribed an appropriate dose of these agents in oral form to prevent the reoccurrence of the side effect.

WHAT KINDS OF MEDICATIONS ARE USED TO TREAT MOOD SYMPTOMS?

Mood stabilizers are used to treat manic mood symptoms that are a component of schizoaffective disorder.

A manic mood is manifested by a highly elevated mood, increased output of speech, increased impulsivity and sometimes grandiose delusions. Mood stabilizers such as lithium and divalproic acid (Depakote, Depakote SR, Depakote ER) are very useful. Antipsychotics are often added to treat manic mood states, especially if there are psychotic symptoms.

If depressive mood symptoms occur, antidepressants can be helpful. There are different types of antidepressants. Those belonging to the selective serotonin reuptake inhibitors (SSRI) class are often helpful.

This SSRI class of antidepressants includes agents such as Fluoxetine (Prozac)

Paroxetine (Paxil)

Sertraline (Zoloft)

Citalopram (Celexa)

Escitalopram (Lexapro)

Antidepressants such as venlafaxine (Effexor XR) and mirtazapine (Remeron) can also be very helpful. Remeron has a side effect of promoting sleep and appetite. This side effect is used for a therapeutic purpose in conditions where poor appetite and insomnia are problematic.

One needs to be aware that antidepressants in schizoaffective disorder, bipolar type and in bipolar disorder can sometimes lead to agitation by activating manic symptoms.

The key to resolving this complication of emerging mania is to stop the antidepressant and add a mood stabilizer such as lithium, Depakote or carbamazepine.

WHAT ARE SOME EFFECTIVE MOOD STABILIZERS?

The following are proven and effective mood stabilizers:

Divalproic Acid (Depakote, Depakote ER): This is an effective mood stabilizer for stabilizing bipolar disorder or schizoaffective disorder bipolar type. It is sometimes used to control aggressive behaviors in individuals with brain injuries. There are no therapeutic levels for treatment use in psychiatry. Levels above 100 should be avoided but sometimes levels up to 120 are needed. Periodic monitoring of liver function and blood levels is recommended, especially when used at the higher doses. There is no defined lower therapeutic level and sometimes a low dose of even 500 mgs is helpful.

There is a risk in some individuals for an elevation of ammonia. The risk may be higher in women. If the individual on Depakote appears unusually sedated or appears confused, it may be a good idea to check their ammonia level. If this is elevated, the mood stabilizing dose can be lowered, or the mood stabilizer can be changed. Lactulose is sometimes added to reduce the ammonia levels.

The typical dose is between 500 and 2000 mg per day. The Depakote ER is convenient to use as it can be used once a day, and this increases compliance and hence efficacy for controlling manic symptoms.

Lithium Carbonate, Lithium Citrate: Lithium is an effective mood stabilizer, however it has a narrow window of therapeutic blood level range. If this narrow range is exceeded, serious side effects can occur. It has to, therefore, be prescribed carefully. The doctor will monitor levels and other labs such as kidney function and thyroid functioning. Thyroid hormone production can be suppressed in individuals who are prescribed lithium. It may also prolong cardiac conduction, and an EKG is recommended to rule out any cardiac contraindications to its use.

Carbamazepine (Tegretol): This is a tricky mood stabilizer to use as it can affect its own metabolism and the metabolism of many other medications whose levels may be lowered when Tegretol is co-prescribed with them. The usual target dose is 600 to 1200 mgs. Periodic Tegretol levels are monitored along with cbc, cmp and a urinalysis.

An EKG may also be indicated as it has a tricyclic structure that can affect cardiac conduction.

WHAT IS HYPONATREMIA (LOW BLOOD SODIUM LEVELS) AND WHY SHOULD IT BE TREATED?

Hyponatremia is a clinical condition of low sodium that can occur as a side effect of medication or due to a unique behavior found in schizophrenia called polydipsia.

Polydipsia is the excessive drinking of water. Sometimes the amount of water drunk is huge. The condition causes a severe dilution of the electrolytes with resultant hyponatremia (low sodium in the blood stream). An excessive dilution and excessive hyponatremia can lead to seizures and death.

The condition needs to be therefore detected early and treated in a very organized and proficient manner. It requires the highest level of competency by the psychiatry and medical staff.

Sometimes medications such as carbamazepine, mentioned above, may also lead to low sodium levels due to a side effect called SIADH (Syndrome of Inappropriate Antidiuretic Hormone).

The ADH, or antidiuretic hormone, is a hormone secreted by a part of the brain called the hypothalamus. When a person is trying to exist in conditions of water drought, such as in a desert, and the water intake is poor due to the scarcity of water, the brain secretes this hormone to stop the diuresis (secretion of water through urine) to avoid dehydration and death. It is a lifesaving mechanism that is triggered by increased concentration of the blood due to unquenched thirst. The body holds back the water that would otherwise have been passed into the urine.

Some medications such as carbamazepine can cause an inappropriate secretion of this hormone, hence the name SIADH side effect. The net result is that an excess of water is retained by the kidneys causing a dilution of the blood stream with a resultant fall in the sodium levels.

The cause of low sodium levels can be hard to discern sometimes. A sodium level below 125 carries increasing risk of seizures and deaths have occurred due to this condition caused by polydipsia.

It becomes important, therefore, for the clinician to figure out the cause.

The urine concentration can usually help to distinguish this. In polydipsia, the urine is dilute as the body recognizes that an excess of water is being drunk and tries to put it out as much as possible, leading to a dilute urine; in SIADH, the body is falsely thinking that it is dying of thirst and retains much more water, leading to a concentration of the urine. The specific gravity of the urine thus tells the tale.

The treatment approaches can be radically different.

The treatment of SIADH begins with discontinuation of the offending agent. In the case of Tegretol that is being used as a mood stabilizer, it can be replaced with Depakote. A cross-tapering with valproic acid (Depakote ER) can help to resolve the problem if the hyponatremia is due to SIADH.

If the low sodium is due to polydipsia, the patient needs to be placed on a 1:1 watch to avoid polydipsia and the water intake needs to be restricted to 2 to 3 liters at the most until the plasma electrolytes normalize, including the concentration of sodium. The medical team should avoid too rapid a correction of the hyponatremia. A hasty correction can lead to neurological damage.

To treat polydipsia, a trial of a different antipsychotic agents such as clozapine can be helpful sometimes in decreasing polydipsia behavior. It is well known in psychiatry to be a difficult condition to treat.

Patients with polydipsia tend to be refractory at some level to antipsychotics. There seems to be some anxiety related exacerbation of the condition as well. Stressful news associated with interpersonal loss seems to trigger an increase in polydipsia behaviors. The psychodynamics of the polydipsia are therefore complex. There are contributing factors from both the psychotic and neurotic domains.

WHAT ARE SOME MEDICATIONS THAT CAN CAUSE SIADH AND LOW SODIUM LEVELS?

There are many medications that have been implicated. Some of these medications are as follows:

- Carbamazepine

- SSRI antidepressants such as fluoxetine, fluvoxamine, paroxetine, and sertraline

  * This SIADH side effect due to SSRIs may be higher in those over age 65

- Tricyclic antidepressants

- Phenothiazine antipsychotics

- Oxytocin

- Prostaglandin inhibitors

- Lisinopril and other ACE inhibitors

- Chlorpropamide

- Cyclophosphamide

- Vincristine

- Some drugs of abuse such as ecstasy and nicotine have also been associated with SIADH.

- The mechanism of how they cause the SIADH effect is not always clear.

HOW LONG DOES IT TAKE TO SEE A BENEFIT FROM ANTIPSYCHOTIC MEDICATIONS?

The benefit can be seen as early as one week. Within five to six weeks, there is a significant remission of psychotic symptoms in a majority of the patients. For patients with schizoaffective disorder who have a manic or depressive component, the time period for response is also rapid, within days to a few weeks.

WHAT ARE SOME SIDE EFFECTS FROM MEDICATIONS USED TO TREAT SCHIZOPHRENIA AND SCHIZOAFFECTIVE DISORDER?

Each medication has its unique side effect profile. With antipsychotics, however, different side effects can sometimes occur. Most of the side effects are treatable or can be minimized. The side effects are as follows:

- Tremors

- Drooling

- Tardive dyskinesia

- Metabolic syndrome

- Acute muscle stiffness also called acute dystonia

Acute dystonia can be distressful and can be rapidly treated by an intramuscular (IM) injection of Benadryl 50 mg IM or Cogentin 2 mgs IM. Taking these doses orally by mouth will also provide relief but will take a bit longer.

These side effects can also be decreased by an adjustment of the dose, changing the medication, or adding medications such as Cogentin or Benadryl that prevent these side effects.

Acute Dystonia is preventable

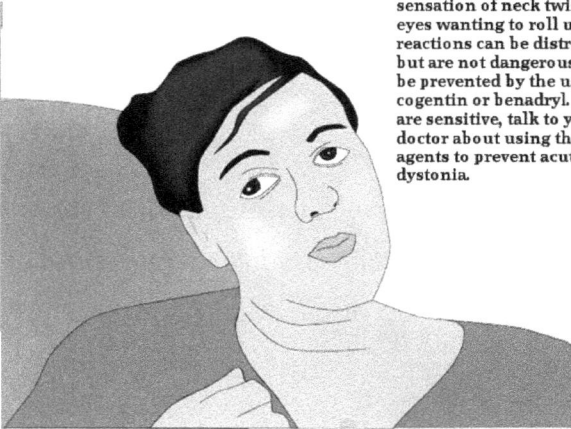

Acute Dystonia is a spasm of a muscle group due to some antipsychotic medications such as haldol, prolixin or others. It can cause a sensation of neck twisting or eyes wanting to roll up. Such reactions can be distressful but are not dangerous. It can be prevented by the use of cogentin or benadryl. If you are sensitive, talk to your doctor about using these agents to prevent acute dystonia.

First, an attempt can be made, if possible, to decrease the dose of the antipsychotic. However, this is not always feasible.

The other option for treating eps (extrapyramidal) or the muscular side effects is to add a standing order of anticholinergic medications like benztropine (Cogentin), Trihexyphenidyl (Artane), or diphenhydramine (Benadryl). Benztropine (Cogentin) 1 to 2 mg two to three times a day or diphenhydramine (Benadryl) 25 to 50 mg two to three times a day. Artane 2 to 4 mg two to three times a day may also be used. It has a unique activating property that may be useful in preventing depression in individuals with comorbid or coexisting depressive symptoms. Some patients may find the effects addictive and may seek out the use of Artane.

An attempt should be made to use lower doses of these medications as they have their own set of side effects such as dry mouth, blurred vision, constipation, and urinary hesitation. These side effects can be particularly problematic in the elderly.

Amantadine (Symmetrel) is sometimes used for the tremor and other motor movement side effects as it does not have the above side effects related to anticholinergics such as Cogentin or Benadryl causing dry mouth, constipation, urinary hesitation and blurred vision. It does, however, have some dopamine stimulating properties and may at times increase psychotic symptoms.

Other Side Effects of Antipsychotic Medications:

In women, by blocking dopamine receptors in the hypothalamus, antipsychotics may cause menstrual irregularities.

Over the long term, there is a risk for abnormal involuntary movements of one or more of the following muscle groups: facial muscles, tongue, trunk, and limbs. This condition is called tardive dyskinesia (TD).

There is no good treatment for this. Sometimes, TD gets better once the medications are stopped. If the patient still needs an antipsychotic for control of psychotic symptoms, clozapine

(Clozaril/Fazaclo) is utilized. The use of clozapine can decrease TD symptoms, sometimes to a significant extent.

Many antipsychotic and antimanic agents, as well as some antidepressants, can cause sedation or sleepiness. If this side effect is experienced, the person should not drive or operate dangerous machinery.

The side effect of sleepiness and drowsiness may decrease as the individual gets used to the medication.

Certain antipsychotics such as Thorazine or quetiapine, clozapine are prone to causing dizziness when first begun and need to be started at a low dose and gradually raised to the effective dose. With other antipsychotics as well, large initial doses can cause dizziness upon rising or changing positions. The key is to get up slowly and in stages, sometimes sitting on the edge of the bed for a minute before rising to a standing position.

Antipsychotics can sometimes cause photosensitivity. This is a condition where the patient develops a rash on areas of skin exposed to sunlight.

Atypical antipsychotics such as olanzapine have been associated with weight gain, an increase in cholesterol and diabetes mellitus. It is important to monitor weight and also check fasting blood sugar levels and lipid levels in an individual taking atypical antipsychotic medications.

One of the distressful side effects of antipsychotic medication is akathisia. This is a sense of continued restlessness when the individual is on an antipsychotic.

This can be treated by adding propranolol (Inderal) in a low dose of 10 mg two to three times a day and titrating the dose to achieve remission of the symptoms. Blood pressure and pulse should be checked as the medication can lower blood pressure and decrease the pulse rate.

Other strategies are to decrease the dose or to switch the antipsychotic. If this is not feasible, other interventions can include the addition of an anticholinergic medication such as benztropine 1mg two to three times a day or addition of antianxiety medication lorazepam 1mg two to three times a day. The lorazepam (Ativan) should be used with caution as it has some addiction risk and can have the side effect of increasing drowsiness.

Getting help for Side Effects

If you experience any side effects from your medication, talk to your doctor. Oftentimes a reduction in the dose of the medication, addition of other meds for the side effect or change of medication can decrease and even eliminate the side effect. If there are any side effects, be sure to tell your doctor.

Many of the side effects decrease after a few weeks on their own as well.

How common is anxiety in schizophrenia and schizoaffective disorder?

Anxiety is common in individuals who suffer from schizophrenia and schizoaffective disorder. This anxiety is different from paranoia. Paranoia is a more pervasive state of mind tied to feeling threatened or persecuted. Anxieties are situational and related to the day-to-day difficulties of coping with voices that are on the increase or difficulties in communicating with others. When anxiety is not resolved, it tends to amplify the underlying paranoia.

WHAT IS AKATHISIA AND HOW CAN IT BE TREATED?

AKATHISIA
(Inability
to Rest)

Akathisia is a side effect that may be falsly diagnosed as worsening psychosis and the dose of antipsychotic may be raised leading to further worsening of this problem.

The treatment is
1. To add one or more of the following:
cogentin, diphenhydramine, propranolol or lorazepam.
2. Consider dose reduction or change of antipsychotic

The person may walk in place, or feel a need to move around

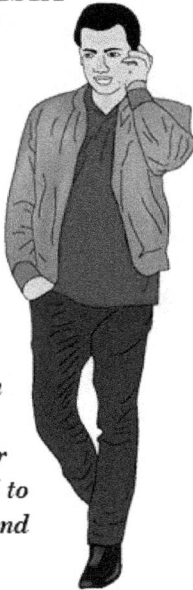

Akathisia is a side effect of certain antipsychotic medications marked by an inability to be at rest. It is often accompanied by a desire to move around, and the person may be observed to be pacing back and forth or even walking in place. It can be stressful and associated with significant anxiety.

Akathisia is very treatable. Relief can be obtained with medications such as propranolol (Inderal) in the dose of 10 to 20mg two to three times a day.

This dose can be titrated up to control the restlessness. Since it is a blood pressure medication also, it can decrease the heart rate and blood pressure resulting in dizziness. It should, therefore, be prescribed under the supervision of a doctor, and vital signs should be taken as needed.

Usually, a low starting dose is not problematic, and the person can achieve a certain state of calm without the distressing need to keep moving.

Other medications such as benztropine and Ativan can also be helpful for akathisia.

This side effect is often easy to miss by the untrained observer. When recognized and treated, it provides significant relief.

Other anxiety states can also coexist with schizophrenia and schizoaffective disorder. Some of these other illnesses include social phobia, PTSD, and obsessive-compulsive disorder. Specific treatments are available for these when they are present. It should be kept in mind, however, that they need to be carefully teased apart from the anxiety and paranoia that is prevalent in schizophrenia and schizoaffective disorder.

Polypharmacy, or use of excessive medications, should be avoided when possible, and the overarching illness of schizophrenia or schizoaffective disorder should be first treated to an optimal degree.

If residual anxiety symptoms exist, individual psychotherapy and psychosocial interventions may also be helpful.

There are, however, certain anxiety states such as OCD that respond only to SSRI medications in the upper dose ranges. When other symptoms of OCD are noted such as obsessions, rituals, and compulsions, such medications provide significant relief of the symptoms.

Anxiety states have a vast differential diagnosis, and this should be looked into in order to rule out any medical or substance abuse-related causes of anxiety.

Medical causes of anxiety can be present even in individuals with schizophrenia and schizoaffective disorder. These organic causes should be treated in their own right if they exist.

WHAT ARE SOME BIO-PSYCHO-SOCIAL TREATMENTS FOR SCHIZOPHRENIA AND SCHIZOAFFECTIVE DISORDER?

The biological treatments, of course, are interventions with medications.

The psychosocial treatments are those that help by providing individual therapy, group therapy, and art therapy. Any measures that foster supportive relationships can also be considered psychosocial in nature. Work with family involving education or answering questions can also be considered a psychosocial intervention.

Psychosocial treatments can also include case management, helping with financial aid, and assistance with social welfare programs.

Schizophrenia, schizoaffective disorder and major mood illnesses such as bipolar disorder tend to be chronic and debilitating, and many individuals are unable to navigate the sea of bureaucracy that lies between them and the benefits they need and are entitled to.

The clinician and the case manager can play an important role in helping to get this done for the patients.

It may be simple as providing contact information for social welfare agencies. Formalized case management services may assist by setting up appointments, arranging transportation and providing other support as needed.

The role of psychosocial interventions cannot be overemphasized. There is no amount of medication that can take the place of the relief provided by the sympathetic ear of a therapist or the comfort of a warm place to stay in the winter.

It is important for the social worker, the psychiatrist and the therapist to work in a collaborative manner to achieve the best outcomes for their common patients.

With enough psychosocial supports, some patients may be able to attain an independent living status, attend school or even go to work.

Families should be made aware of how heated arguments and loud conflicts (high expressed emotions) can be detrimental to the well-being of the person who suffers from schizophrenia or schizoaffective disorder.

Families can also be important allies for recovery when they encourage compliance with medications. They should be educated to do so. A simple word or two from a trusted family member about compliance can go a long way.

The patient can also be provided with education about the warning signs of relapse and encouraged to plan in advance what steps to take to avoid a full-blown relapse. Patients can be taught coping skills that can help them decrease anxiety related to their symptoms or other psychosocial difficulties.

The individual can be taught social skills, and this can make it easier for them to get along with others and avoid miscommunications.

Job and vocational training also have a role in the rehabilitation of the individual. This can be a component of psychosocial interventions for higher functioning individuals.

They may also need training in the use of transportation services and in the management of their financial affairs. Simple organizational tips can be a great help.

Counseling in regards to the avoidance of alcohol and substance abuse is also a critical component of psychosocial interventions since this is often tied to problems with the law.

WHAT IS THE ROLE OF COGNITIVE BEHAVIORAL THERAPY IN SCHIZOPHRENIA AND SCHIZOAFFECTIVE DISORDER?

It was taught at one time that psychodynamic and cognitive behavioral therapies were only useful for high functioning individuals with neurotic anxiety and depressive states.

More recent evidence indicates that structured cognitive behavioral therapy can be quite useful for some individuals with psychotic disorders.

They can be allowed to challenge their fears and beliefs through testing and verifying the validity of their fears.

Rational strategies to cope with their stress through relaxation techniques can be taught even if the stress is due to a sense of persecution due to a delusion. The stress is very real for the person and coping skills to deal with the resultant distress can be helpful even if the delusion proves refractory to the medication.

Sometimes, using a mental imagery of visualizing a stop sign when hallucinations occur has been helpful for some patients in lessening the hallucinations or for calming their anxieties.

A person can have a phrase or affirmation that guides them about their safety. This can be a written phrase, or prayer, that they carry on them like a talisman.

Other individuals might find keeping a small Bible or crucifix or other religious protective symbol to be helpful.

The key is to let the individual decide what is comforting to them and to encourage them to use it.

Coping skills can also include meditation, listening to music, talking to a friend, taking a drive or a walk or a visit to the local coffee shop or bookstore.

HOW EASY IS IT TO GET HELP FOR SCHIZOPHRENIA AND SCHIZOAFFECTIVE DISORDER?

Help is easier to obtain in some areas than others. The following options exist in many areas:

1. One can always go to the emergency room if the symptoms are acute in nature.

2. One can check the Yellow Pages or use one of the search engines such as Google to look for psychiatrists that are available in the community.

3. If a person has Medicaid or Medicare or other insurance, there may be a website that shows the names of the doctors and other clinicians that accept your insurance.

4. If there is a large medical center affiliated with a medical training program, they may have a psychiatry department that has clinics where treatment is often provided at an adjusted, lower rate according to the ability to afford such care.

5. Catholic charities and other religious organizations have medical and psychiatry staff affiliated with them. They will often see patients for free. Having worked briefly with them, I can say that they are fine organizations that offer help to the

homeless in many areas other than medical and psychiatric care. They are the best living examples of God's love for the poor and downtrodden amongst us.

6. If you have no insurance and are indigent, you can still go to the emergency room and cannot be denied care.

7. Some state psychiatric hospitals are still open and take walk-ins. This means you can walk into the main entrance and ask for help. They can provide inpatient care and may have partial day programs and outpatient care as well. They can also link you with other resources in the community where you may be able to get help.

8. If you are a veteran, the VA hospitals offer excellent psychiatric services by very qualified psychiatrists. The VA also has many outreach programs for veterans and centers that are located in rural communities to lessen the commute time. The VA provides a full range of services including housing and substance abuse counseling, with inpatient and outpatient psychiatric care. I have worked with the VA and can attest to the quality of their staff. They truly care for the veterans and have a great attitude about providing good care.

WHAT INFORMATION SHOULD I TAKE WITH ME FOR A VISIT WITH THE PSYCHIATRIST?

There is no need to stress out about the visit. All physicians are sworn by the Hippocratic Oath to first do no harm. A psychiatrist is a medical doctor first, with four years of additional training in psychiatry.

The following steps may help you gain more from your visit:

1. You can write down your questions beforehand so that you don't forget to ask something that is important to you.

2. Take a list of the medications that you are taking. Ensure this list also contains any over the counter (OTC) medications that you may be on.

3. It is important to give the complete list so that he can be sure that there are no interactions with any psychiatric medications that he may want to prescribe.

4. Let the doctor know if you smoke cigarettes.

5. Let the doctor know if you use alcohol or drugs and when the last use was.

6. Let the doctor know if any other family member is taking any psychiatric medications.

7. If a certain medication worked well with a blood relative, let the doctor know. This medication may work well for you as well if you suffer from similar symptoms.

8. Arrange for transportation ahead of time.

9. If a family member or friend can accompany you that will be helpful. Having a family member or friend with you can help you get better care.

10. Do not approach the doctor as an adversary and advise your friend or relative of the same. He or she is there to help you.

11. Remember, you cannot be forced to take any medication against your will if you do not pose a threat to yourself or to others.

12. If you think you are a threat to yourself or are having thoughts of harming another person, please call 911 and get yourself to a hospital on a voluntary basis.

13. If you are unable to keep your appointment, it is courteous to call and cancel the appointment and reschedule at another time that is more convenient.

14. If you have a history of allergy or severe adverse effect from a medication, let your doctor know.

15. Let him or her know if you are experiencing any adverse side effects.

16. Let the doctor know what coping strategies you use to deal with any stress. This may be walking, art therapy, listening to music etc.

SHOULD I AVOID THE USE OF ALCOHOL AND ILLICIT DRUGS THAT I HAVE USED FOR RECREATIONAL PURPOSES?

Yes, it is a very good idea to abstain from the use of alcohol and definitely to abstain from the use of any illicit drugs. They can worsen the course of your illness and increase the risk of adverse side effects from the medications or render them ineffective. Some psychiatric medications are sedating and this combined with alcohol or other sedating street drugs can lead to a dangerous level of sedation or respiratory suppression and death.

WHAT ARE THE KEYS TO STAYING WELL IF YOU HAVE SCHIZOPHRENIA?

Keys to Long Term Recovery From Schizophrenia and Schizoaffective Disorder

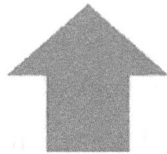

Supportive Empathic Relationships

1. **Psychosocial Treatments**
2. **Supportive Therapy**
3. **Medication Compliance**
4. **Depot Medications**

Depot Medications are medications that can be injected once every 2 to 4 weeks. Examples are Haldol Decanoate, Prolixin Decanoate, Risperdal Consta, etc.

The keys are as follows:

1. Take your medications.

2. Go to your appointments. If you miss an appointment, call and reschedule it.

3. Avoid the use of alcohol or drugs.

4. Avoid loud arguments and loud, critical people.

5. Make a friend or a family member your ally or "go to person" to sound off your concerns and to help you advocate for your needs when necessary.

6. Join a support group if one is available in your community.

7. Avoid the company of those who use drugs or are noncompliant with drugs. If possible, encourage them to take their medications and to avoid the use of alcohol or drugs.

8. Ask your doctor to make your medications once a day or twice a day only. Once a day is preferable.

9. Put your medications next to your toothbrush or your keys so that you are reminded daily to take them when you go out or perform the normal activities of daily living such as brushing your teeth.

10. Ask for a long acting injection of the antipsychotic if you have trouble taking your oral medications on a regular basis. This will reduce the risk for relapse and also simplify your life in other ways.

WHAT ARE THE ADVANTAGES OF TAKING A LONG ACTING INJECTABLE ANTIPSYCHOTIC?

The advantages are as follows:

1. A more even and steady level of the antipsychotic is achieved.

2. This may allow for an overall lower level of antipsychotic that is required to control the symptoms.

3. The risk for side effects is lessened.

4. It significantly decreases the relapse risk.

WHAT IS THE NORMAL COURSE OF THE SCHIZOPHRENIA AND SCHIZOAFFECTIVE DISORDER?

The normal course varies but is generally hopeful.

1. About 42 percent of people may have a first episode that meets the criteria but then go into remission and never have another episode again. It is important to remind the individual newly diagnosed with schizophrenia of this positive outlook as many of them become dismayed and disheartened by the illness. There is a false perception that a diagnosis of schizophrenia means the cancelation all major life goals and aspirations. This is definitely not the case given that 42 percent go into remission never to have the symptoms again, and many of the other individuals with schizophrenia can be treated effectively.

2. About 30 percent have significant relief of symptoms, but some mild to moderate symptoms may remain.

3. The remaining 30 percent may have moderate to severe symptoms that may need trials of different medications and Clozaril if the symptoms prove to be refractory. With Clozaril, many more patients find relief from their symptoms.

4. Those in the last category may require more support and placement in supervised settings such as a group home or a hospital setting.

In summary, about 70 percent can lead an almost normal life with the help of good treatment.

HOW FREQUENT IS DEPRESSION IN INDIVIDUALS WHO HAVE SCHIZOPHRENIA?

This is a good question because schizophrenia does sometimes exist with a coexisting depression. It is often overlooked because of the following reasons:

1. The negative symptoms of schizophrenia such as social withdrawal and lack of initiative due to the features of avolition can look like depression. This is because clinical depression is also manifested by social withdrawal, and a certain lethargy and lack of initiative. If a person is depressed and has schizophrenia, and this does happen, it may go unnoticed because the latter symptoms of depression may be confused with the negative symptoms of schizophrenia— namely the avolition and withdrawal symptoms of schizophrenia.

2. There is a flattening of the affect in schizophrenia. This is basically a lack of emotional responsiveness. The person does not have associated sadness.

   In depression, there is also a lack of emotional expressiveness. In depression, however, there is always some sense of sadness, worthlessness, and pessimism about the future. At times, there may be suicidal ideations.

Depression in individuals with schizophrenia may be missed because a decrease in emotional expression is a normal part of the illness of schizophrenia. There are, however, no features such as hopelessness, or worthlessness accompanying schizophrenia.

If such themes are found, a coexisting state of depression is the cause and should be treated. It is a good idea to ask about depression and the symptoms that are associated with depression during every visit with the patient.

The patient should also feel free to report any significant feelings of depression, worthlessness or any thoughts of self-harm or suicide. Medications can rapidly treat the symptoms so that the mood improves and the person can lead a more fulfilling life despite the illness.

3. The parkinsonian side effects of many of the antipsychotic medications cause a masklike face and decreased emotional expressiveness. The doctor may misinterpret the constricted affect and sadness to be parkinsonian side effects of the medications that the person with schizophrenia is taking. and not a feature of underlying sadness or depression.

If the parkinsonian side effects are treated, the underlying sadness and constriction of affect may be more noticeable.

Studies indicate that rates of depression are significant in some individuals with schizophrenia. If thoughts of suicide, worthlessness or hopelessness emerge, these should be reported at the earliest time possible to the treating doctor so that antidepressant medications may be prescribed to treat the depression.

In addition to the medications, depression can also be helped by individual therapy, group therapy, and other psychosocial measures.

WHAT IS A MANIC SWITCH?

When individuals with depression are placed on antidepressants, they may go from being depressed to normal to being elated and manic. This is more likely to occur if there is an underlying bipolar disorder or schizoaffective disorder bipolar type. The manic switch may be a higher risk with tricyclic antidepressants and higher doses of venlafaxine (Effexor).

It is important to watch out for this, and if it should it occur, the antidepressant should be withdrawn and a mood stabilizer such as lithium, Depakote or carbamazepine added to control the manic symptoms.

HOW DOES SCHIZOPHRENIA AFFECT FAMILY MEMBERS?

Family members may be saddened by the illness and be baffled by the symptoms that it produces. They should, however, not blame the person with the illness but accept the fact that the illness does occur and that it is not anyone's fault.

Family members should support each other and the sick family member. Loud, interpersonal arguments and blaming of any one person should be avoided at all costs.

The head of the family, or some designated family member who has read about the illness, should explain how the illness may interfere with the ability to organize self-care and planning in the individual.

Support with making appointments and activities of daily living may be needed while the person recovers from the acute phase of an illness or a relapse.

HOW CAN ONE GET MEDICATIONS ON THE CHEAP IF ONE DOES NOT HAVE INSURANCE COVERAGE?

Several pharmacies have discount plans where you can get a month's supply of many medications for 4 to 5 dollars. These are good generic medications whose purity and authenticity has been verified. The generic medications are reliable and undergo certain tests to ensure their quality.

Affordable medications can be a great relief for individuals who have no insurance. The cost of brand name medications can run into hundreds of dollars.

The website below has information about many medications that are available with a cost of only 4 dollars for a month's supply.

http://www.walmart.com/cp/1078664?povid=5431+%7C+contentZone1+%7C+2014-11-01+%7C+1+%7C+LN-Value+4+Dollar+Prescriptions

Some of the meds listed are as follows:

$4 for a 30-day Supply

$10 for a 90-day Supply

Amitriptyline 10mg

30 tablets

90 tablets

Amitriptyline 25mg

30 tablets

90 tablets

Amitriptyline 50mg

30 tablets

90 tablets

Amitriptyline 75mg

30 tablets

90 tablets

Amitriptyline 100mg

30 tablets

90 tablets

Benztropine 2mg

30 tablets

90 tablets

Buspirone 5mg

60 tablets

180 tablets

Buspirone 10mg*

60 tablets

180 tablets

Citalopram 20mg

30 tablets

90 tablets

Citalopram 40mg

30 tablets

90 tablets

Fluphenazine 1mg

30 tablets

90 tablets

Haloperidol 0.5mg

30 tablets

90 tablets

Haloperidol 1mg

30 tablets

90 tablets

Haloperidol 2mg

30 tablets

90 tablets

Haloperidol 5mg

30 tablets

90 tablets

Lithium Carbonate 300mg*

90 capsules

270 capsules

Nortriptyline 10mg*

30 capsules

90 capsules

Nortriptyline 25mg*

30 capsules

90 capsules

Paroxetine 10mg*

30 tablets

90 tablets

Paroxetine 20mg*

30 tablets

90 tablets

Prochlorperazine 10mg

30 tablets

90 tablets

Trazodone 50mg

30 tablets

90 tablets

Trazodone 100mg

30 tablets

90 tablets

Trazodone 150mg

30 tablets

Trihexyphenidyl 2mg

60 tablets

180 tablets

Other pharmacies such as Walgreens or Rite Aid also have prescription programs similar to this. It is a good idea to ask your local pharmacist for more information in this regard.

CHAPTER 5

OTHER TOPICS OF INTEREST

FACTORS ASSOCIATED WITH VIOLENCE

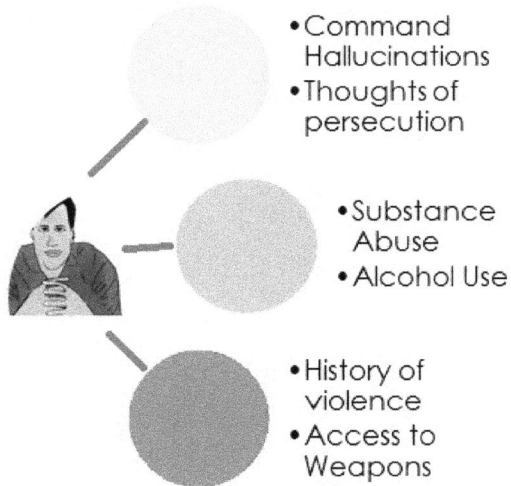

- Command Hallucinations
- Thoughts of persecution

- Substance Abuse
- Alcohol Use

- History of violence
- Access to Weapons

ARE PEOPLE WITH SCHIZOPHRENIA OR SCHIZOAFFECTIVE DISORDER VIOLENT?

People with schizophrenia and schizoaffective disorder are, by nature, likely to seek solitude and are in general not a higher risk for violence.

Most violent crimes, in fact, are the work of criminals who do not suffer from mental illness.

It is important to consider a few factors, however, when making a treatment plan to reduce the risk of violence. In cases where violence occurs, one or more of the following factors may exist:

- A lack of compliance with medications

- A history of violence

- Ongoing alcohol or substance abuse problems

WHAT ARE SOME WAYS OF PREVENTING VIOLENCE TOWARDS FAMILY MEMBERS?

Family members are the most common victims of violence by patients who suffer from schizophrenia or schizoaffective disorder. This is because they often live near the patient, and may become complacent about the warning signs of decompensation.

At other times, they may interact in a manner that is condescending and unsupportive or is perceived in that manner by the patient.

The risk of violence can be reduced by taking the following steps:

1. Ensuring compliance with treatment

2. Addressing of any side effects early to increase compliance

3. Use of Depot, long-acting antipsychotics to increase compliance with treatment

4. Education about consequences of violence

5. Anger Management and CBT to help in coping with sense of persecution without resorting to violence

6. Abstinence from Alcohol

7. Abstinence from Stimulant Drugs, PCP or any other mind-altering drugs

8. Removal of weapons from the home

9. Separation and hospitalization for acute exacerbations early by recognizing prodromal signs and early signs of relapse

10. Anticipating possible problems in the future and defining a plan ahead of time for coping with the problem. These steps should be clearly outlined

WHAT ARE SOME WAYS TO PROMOTE GOOD MENTAL HEALTH?

This is a far-ranging topic, and everyone has their own take on this. It is helpful to keep some of the following ideas in mind when thinking of promoting good mental health:

When we let the person know in word and deed that he or she is valued, it is conducive to promoting good mental health. The value or worth of the person should not be restricted to their achievements or abilities.

A life in which the person feels relatively secure promotes good mental health.

A sense of right and wrong and fostering of empathy for others is helpful in building a stable personality pattern in childhood. This promotes attitudes that are prosocial and adaptive.

The absence of alcohol and substance use is conducive to good mental health.

Exercise and attention to maintaining good physical health are conducive to good mental health.

Having long-term, supportive relationships is conducive to good mental health.

A strong faith or belief in a benign, loving higher power is conducive to good mental health.

A good marriage can be a blessing and promotes wellbeing.

Strong, supportive relationships are associated with better physical health, better emotional health and a greater longevity of life.

DO BLIND PEOPLE EXPERIENCE HALLUCINATIONS?

Yes, a syndrome of Lilliputian hallucinations occurs in blind patients sometimes. These are hallucinations of small and miniature people and animals that are seen to be moving around the room.

The blind individual recognizes that these are hallucinations. These are benign in nature and do not indicate the presence of schizophrenia.

WHAT IS THE ROLE OF NATURE VS. NURTURE IN CAUSING SCHIZOPHRENIA?

Schizophrenia and related psychotic illnesses get precipitated in the context of a biological predisposition. This biological disposition, when exposed to certain environmental stressors, can precipitate a state of altered reality and psychosis.

This process is similar to the predisposition of a person with a strong family history of diabetes to becoming a diabetic when environmental factors such as obesity, and a sedentary lifestyle are present. For schizophrenia and schizoaffective disorder, if there is a genetic predisposition, the exposure to certain environmental factors such as specific infections, head injuries, childhood abuse and neglect may increase the risk. In fact, 40 to 60 percent of the risk may be environmental.

WHAT IS THE ROLE OF BIRTH MONTH AND SCHIZOPHRENIA?

One of the recurring themes is the role of the seasonality of birth and the various environmental factors present at certain times of the year that may be underlying such a seasonality. To be more specific, it has been noted in multiple studies that schizophrenia patients tend to have higher rates of birth during the late winter and early spring.

Some thoughts on this are as follows:

1. Over the eons, schizophrenia has changed at times in its symptom pattern due to the subtle but far-reaching interactions between the developing brain with mutating infectious agents. Catatonic schizophrenia, so common in the wards of state hospitals a century ago, is hardly seen anymore. In its place, the incidence of schizoaffective disorder seems to be much higher.

2. The influenza virus is one of the infectious agents implicated in schizophrenia causation. Its seasonal pattern is felt to be related in some way to a higher incidence of schizophrenia in children born in late winter and the early spring months.

3. Influenza is known to change its genotype (genetic code) with every season such that new vaccine sets have to be created.

Such genetic drift over time may cause a variation in how it interacts with the developing brain and the resultant illness it creates.

Given this, it is likely that schizophrenia symptoms in the future will change in some ways.

WHY DO MUTATIONS OCCUR IN NATURE AND WHY DOES MENTAL ILLNESS EVOLVE OVER TIME?

Nature seems to be testing the limits of our possibilities by perpetually tinkering with its crown jewel—the human brain. This tinkering process may create madness or genius. With genius, humanity takes giant steps forward that uniform, normal, human beings would not have been able to take.

Perhaps the two, madness and genius, are akin after all. It is no wonder that some of the close relatives of brilliant scientists such as Einstein and Nash were diagnosed with schizophrenia as well. They shared the same set of genes being true sons of their great fathers.

Schizophrenia is an illness that touches the essence of what it means to be human—our very own thought processes.

While some faiths have demonized the symptoms of this illness, other religious faiths have recognized this sacred ground and honored the illness and those afflicted as being touched by something special. Provisions have been made for the humane treatment of the mentally ill in such enlightened cultures.

The fact that schizophrenia incidence of one percent is fairly stable and persistent across the world, despite attempts to sterilize it (literally) out of existence by some countries, indicates some essential value in the vulnerability to this illness we call schizophrenia or "split mind".

Evolutionary behaviorists have theorized that a brain that is vulnerable to such alteration of thought provides a potential for madness but also perhaps for the genius that can take humankind forward into new paradigms much as Einstein did in the beginning of the last century. It is, perhaps, the genes for schizophrenia that led him to devise his "thought experiments" that provided him insights into the unity of matter and energy and into the relativity of time.

DOES MENTAL ILLNESS AFFECT THE INTELLIGENCE OF A PERSON?

The intelligence of the person is not affected by their mental illness. It does not lower their IQ. With chronic mental illness, there is some decrease in the working memory and some decrease in the speed of data processing in some patients. This, however, is not significant, and the individual can compensate by increasing attention, taking notes and using organizational strategies.

IS IT POSSIBLE TO PREVENT SCHIZOPHRENIA?

There are many different factors that are associated with the risk for development of schizophrenia. Some factors may yet be unknown, and no one factor is the ultimate cause of the illness.

Some of these factors include the unique genetic code every human is born with. Other factors include the possible exposure to certain infections at a vulnerable period. Yet other factors indicate an association with low birth weight and premature birth.

The use of illicit drugs or alcohol by the mother and the stress level of the mother have also been implicated. Other factors may include any history of physical and emotional trauma or abuse during childhood. The truth of the matter is that we do not know how one or more of these factors interact to produce the unique syndromes of schizophrenia.

The type of relationship that the person has with his or her parents or spouse can have a positive or negative effect on the manifestations of the illness. Since so many factors go into the risk for these illnesses, it is not really possible to give specific advice about the prevention of this illness. To the extent possible, any risk factor that can be decreased should be decreased.

CAN SCHIZOPHRENIA RISK BE LESSENED IN A FUTURE CHILD WHEN ONE OR BOTH PARENTS HAVE SCHIZOPHRENIA?

Risk for Inheritance of Schizophrenia

When One Parent Has Schizophrenia	When Both Parents Have Schizophrenia
14 Percent	40 Percent

One of the unique ideas proposed for prevention of schizophrenia if one or both of the parents have schizophrenia is as follows:

1. Use of a contraceptive method during the months of May, June, July and August if the mother lives in the Northern Hemisphere. This birth control can be achieved with oral contraceptives or other techniques.

2. Since many of the birth months for individuals with schizophrenia and schizoaffective disorder tend to be late winter or early spring, it is possible that the risk could be lessened if the pregnancy is avoided nine months earlier. This

would mean strict birth control during the months of May to August. This may decrease the risk of exposure to infections that seem to be associated with higher rates of schizophrenia in babies born in late winter and early spring.

3. A similar strategy could be devised for the Southern Hemisphere as well with the use of contraception during the months of October, November, December, and January. The seasonality of birth month in the Southern Hemisphere, however, has less robust data than that of the Northern Hemisphere. That does not mean it does not exist.

For a mother or father who has schizophrenia and wants to become a parent, it is a strategy worth considering to lower the risk of schizophrenia in their child.

What Other Measures Can Be Taken To Decrease The Risk Of Schizophrenia In A Child Who Has A Higher Genetic Risk For Schizophrenia?

The following steps may decrease the risk:

Once the mother is pregnant, she should be provided a loving and supportive home atmosphere. The use of alcohol and drugs should be avoided. Antenatal care visits should be scheduled to ensure the physical health of the mother and child.

Once the child is born, he or she should be provided with a loving and supportive atmosphere wherein he or she is made to feel accepted and appreciated. The parent should be warm and engaged and avoid an ambivalent and distant relationship. Emotional reciprocation with games such as peek-a-boo and others may lay down correct emotional connectivity between thought and emotions.

It seems that the childhood of some schizophrenic patients had a degree of emotional sterility. This may be reflective of parental attitudes that embody a level of cold intellectuality that steals the warmth in a relationship. This lack of warm, emotional expressivity in parents or caretakers may be a risk factor that disrupts easy correlations and connection between emotions and thoughts in the young, developing brain. By using some play activity that allows for the expression of emotions in a warm, joyful play, it may be possible to decrease the risk for the emergence of the split mind or schizophrenia that cannot associate thought and emotions, or schizophrenia, in later life.

WHAT IS SPLIT PERSONALITY AND HOW IS IT DIFFERENT FROM SCHIZOPHRENIA AND SCHIZOAFFECTIVE DISORDER?

Split personality, or multiple personality disorder as it is sometimes called, is a type of post-traumatic state that seems to be caused by a massive suppression of emotionally traumatic memories.

These memories and associated emotions are compartmentalized in different schemas, or emotional "folders" if you will. Sealing off such traumatic turmoil is therapeutic in many ways, and many of us use this consciously or unconsciously. This allows the person to operate effectively to some extent.

In the person with a history of extensive trauma, the brain may not have been able to make sense of the entire series of events. It consequently seals off experiences that do not conform with other experiences of the individual. Within each component of a person's psyche that is sealed off, there is an evolution of an inner logic to retain control of the circumstances associated with that trauma. These responses may be extreme and not totally integrated into the personality of the individual.

These parallel emotional worlds can coexist side by side and be unaware of each other. When new stressors arise, the individual may resort to an earlier pattern of coping that involved a different set of responses.

The shift of paradigms can be sudden and associated with congruent changes in the mannerisms and even the physiology of the individual.

Such dissociative identities are uncommon. Histrionic presentations of what individuals think is "multiple personality" is a more likely phenomeon. Such presentations, however, should also not be scoffed at as they indicate an unmet emotional need for which therapy should be provided.

The other name for Multiple Personality Disorder is Dissociative Identity Disorder.

These individuals do not experience hallucinations and do not suffer from delusions like patients with schizophrenia do.

The split implied in the term schizophrenia is the splitting of emotion from thought. Emotion in psychiatric jargon is called "affect". Bleuler noticed that some persons with schizophrenia might discuss events with significant emotional significance but without expressing the accompanying affect (emotion) such as sadness or happiness. Their faces seemed unexpressive and flat, hence he called this a flat affect. In other words, they had a flat emotional tone during their conversations or inappropriate emotional expressions that did not coincide with what they were verbally expressing.

In a typical mental status exam, a concept called the "range of affect" is used. The range of affect simply means the range of emotional expressions that the individual uses in expressing themselves. These affects include emotions such as joy, anger, or sadness with accompanying emotional expressions and gestures. The affect in schizophrenia becomes blunted to different degrees.

The person, for example, may exhibit laughter or may smile when he or she is describing a sad event that should be accompanied by expressions of sadness, grief or sorrow.

WHICH MEMBER OF THE TREATMENT TEAM IS ESSENTIAL FOR TREATING SCHIZOPHRENIA AND SCHIZOAFFECTIVE DISORDER?

In one sense, the optimal treatment of the individual requires a team approach, hence no one member of the team is more important than the other. In another sense, in terms of training, a well-trained psychiatrist is essential when it comes to treating these disorders. He has a global perspective including the biological and pharmacological knowledge required to treat those with mental illnesses such as schizophrenia and schizoaffective disorder.

The formulation of a good treatment plan depends on and is predicated on making an accurate diagnosis. A trained psychiatrist should be able to diagnose schizophrenia with a fair degree of certainty. Other mental health professionals such as a doctor of psychology are also qualified to recognize the major signs and symptoms. Before a diagnosis can be finalized, however, it is important that potential medical causes of the symptoms are ruled out. Since a psychiatrist is the only member of the team trained as a medical doctor, he is better qualified to understand the role of medical disorders and should, therefore, make the final diagnosis.

WHO ARE SOME FAMOUS INDIVIDUALS THAT HAVE BEEN DIAGNOSED WITH SCHIZOPHRENIA?

There are many such people.

Sometimes, although the individual had features of schizophrenia, they still managed to accomplish great things such as the mathematician John Nash.

The following individuals were diagnosed with schizophrenia during their lifetime. This information is gathered from the public domain, and no confidentiality is breached.

Lionel Aldridge- NFL Player

John Nash- Nobel Prize Winner/Mathematics

Tom Harrel- Jazz Musician

Meera Popkin- Broadway Star

Eduard Einstein- Son of Albert Einstein (Nobel Prize Winner)

Dr. James Watson's son (Dr. Watson co-discovered the DNA structure and won the Nobel Prize)

Alan Alda's mother (Alan Alda was a star of the TV series MASH)

Vaclav Nijinsky- Famous Russian Dancer

Jack Kerouac- Author

Rose Williams- Sister of Author Tennessee Williams

It appears that the vulnerability for schizophrenia may sometimes be associated with great talent in other family members who have excelled in drama, the arts, and innovative sciences.

CHAPTER 6

PSYCHIATRIC GLOSSARY

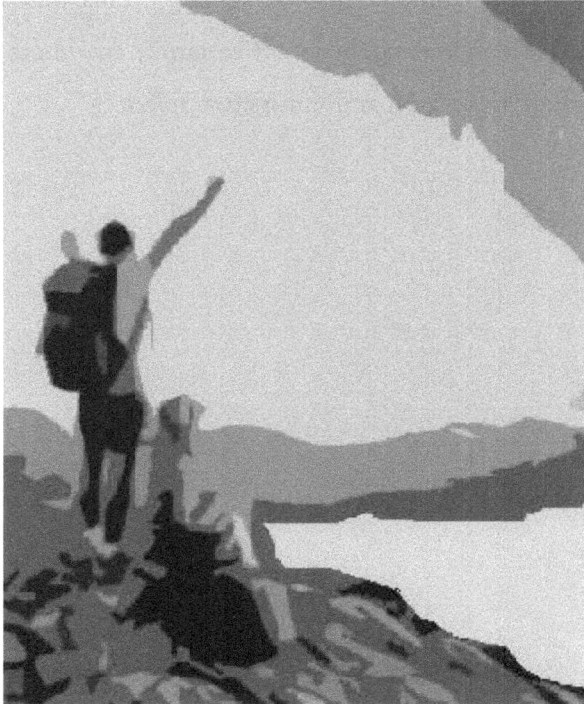

It is important to understand the language of psychiatry. Some words are frequently used and have a precise meaning. It is important to have some understanding of these words. If you are familiar with these, you may skip over this chapter. If you need to check on a word, you can come back to this glossary. This list is not comprehensive, so if you come across a new word that is not on this list, it is a good idea to google it or consult a dictionary. Here are some common psychiatric terms worth understanding.

Abulia: Lack of initiative or will. The person may neglect basic aspects of grooming or hygiene. This may exist in schizophrenia or depressive disorders.

Hyperbulia: Excessive drive or will. This may exist in mania, various impulse control disorders, and paraphilias.

Alogia: A decrease in talking.

Avolition: Lack of initiative in starting tasks. The term has a meaning similar to abulia (lack of will).

Anosognosia: This is the lack of awareness of an illness. The person with a right parietal lobe stroke may deny the existence of the left side of the face and leave that part of the face unshaved. In psychiatry, it refers to the gross lack of insight into the presence of a psychiatric illness.

Affect: This is a unique term in psychiatry. It does not mean effect. The term affect refers to a range of emotional display that accompanies communication between the individual and another person. The range of affect can vary from expressions such as a simple smile, smirk, frown or other expressions of joy to sadness and all emotions in between.

These are conveyed mostly by changing expressions of the face, voice, or body gestures. In schizophrenia, the range of emotional expression is greatly dampened and is said to be flat. The person's expressions come across as flat, hence the affect is called a flat affect. If it constricted due to depression, it is called a constricted affect by an unstated convention. If it is due to psychosis, it is called a flat affect. These can be hard to tell apart sometimes.

A similar flattening or constriction of affect (emotional expressions) may sometimes be the result of cultural indoctrination. Some cultures do encourage the suppression of excessive emotionality. Such expression may be viewed as a sign of disrespect. Individuals in such cultures are encouraged not to be very expressive in front of authority figures as a mark of respect.

At other times, a flat or constricted affect can be linked with the traumatic numbing of emotions due to post-traumatic stress disorder (PTSD). In these conditions, however, there are none of the other features of schizophrenia such as hearing of voices or paranoid or bizarre thought content.

Inappropriate Affect: This is the expression of happiness and laughter when discussing sad things or an appearance of sadness when talking about happy things. The expression is inappropriate to the thought content. Individuals under extreme stress may at times also express an inappropriate affect.

Professor Affect: Inappropriate or flat affect at times can be found in Asperger's syndrome or the "professor syndrome". In real professors and highly intelligent individuals, affect can also appear somewhat "off". The brain seems to go ahead of the expressional speed of the person giving emotions their stilted appearance.

Constricted affect: A restricted range of emotions due to anxiety or depression.

Bipolar Disorder: An illness that has alternating bouts of abnormal elevation of mood or deep levels of depression is called bipolar disorder. In between the two extreme mood states, there is usually a period of normal level mood.

A normal day to day variation of moods does not qualify for bipolar disorder. It must be a persistent, sustained state of abnormally elevated or depressed mood for a defined minimum period of one week in mania and two weeks for depression. The mood duration can be shorter if treated and if there is a history of prior diagnosis of bipolar disorder.

A quick change of emotional expressions from easy crying to laughter when accompanied by other signs such as grandiosity and rapid speech may be a sign of bipolar disorder. A flippant or mercurial attitude related to the personality of a person does not qualify as bipolar disorder.

Affect and Mood: Another way to describe affect in comparison to mood is to use the analogy of weather. Affect is the changing day to day weather, and the Mood of a person is similar to the climate of a region such as a warm climate or a cold climate. If the person is generally depressed most of the days, his mood is said to be depressed; if he or she is in a normal mood they may be sad for a little while over a setback but bounce back. A normal mood is also described as being in a euthymic state. Euthymic means level and normal. If the mood is unusually upbeat, it is described as elevated mood. This is not the situational upbeat mood of a positive event or some good news.

Mood, by definition, is a longer range description. By implying an elevated mood in a person, the clinician is also implying the possibility of bipolar disorder in a person related to manic or hypomanic features.

Mania: Mania is the elevation of mood to a degree that it is dysfunctional. An example would be if the person bankrupted themselves due to their grandiosity and generosity due to an elevated mood.

Hallucination: A sensory experience that occurs in the absence of stimuli in the environment.

Auditory Hallucinations: Hearing voices or sounds when no one is present in the environment. Auditory hallucinations are the most common type of hallucination in schizophrenia and schizoaffective disorder

Visual Hallucinations: Seeing objects, shapes, persons without objective evidence of such stimuli being in the environment. Visual hallucinations if they occur in schizophrenia are uncommon and often fleeting.

Olfactory Hallucination: Sensation of smelling an odor when there is no source of the odor in the environment. This is rare. It is sometimes associated with seizures or tumors in the part of the brain associated with smell perception.

Gustatory Hallucination: It is the sensation of tasting something without the presence of food or drink in the mouth.

Tactile Hallucination: It is the sensation of being touched on the skin in the absence of anyone or anything touching the person.

Formication: It is a special type of tactile hallucinations that is produced in association with the use of stimulants such as cocaine, amphetamines or others. It is described as a sensation of worms crawling under the skin. The person may try to pick them out of the skin causing breaks in the skin. Such "skin picking" lesions are common in heavy users of stimulant drugs.

Illusion: It is the false perception of something based on the misperception of a real object. For example, a rope hanging from a peg is misperceived to be a snake.

Overvalued Ideas: These are peculiar, unique beliefs that the person holds fast to but they are amenable to changing them when presented with strong data to point out a better alternative hypothesis.

Delusions: A false fixed belief that cannot be changed despite irrefutable evidence to the contrary. For example, a man believes devices have been placed in his neck by aliens despite x-rays, CAT scans and MRIs showing that there are no foreign bodies in his neck.

Delusions can be of different types. Some of these are as follows.

Paranoid Delusions: These are false fixed beliefs that someone or something is out to get them and means to do them harm. Delusions of persecution are similar.

Erotomanic Delusions: These are false fixed beliefs that a celebrity or another important person is secretly in love with them or that they have a special relationship with this important person when none exists. Movie stars and celebrities are sometimes stalked by individuals with erotomanic delusions. John Hinckley had an erotomanic delusion centered on Jodie Foster and of having a special love relationship with her. He attempted to forge the bonds of this love further by shooting at President Reagan.

Somatic Delusion: A false fixed belief that there is some defect in the shape or look of a particular body part of the person.

Hypomania: This is an elevation of mood that is to a degree that is less than mania. Hypomania is not dysfunctional. Individuals in a hypomanic state can accomplish much, in fact, and may be star performers. There is always a risk, however, of hypomania going into mania. Antidepressants can do this.

Catatonia: An altered mental state wherein the person may maintain a certain posture for a long period while remaining mute. Like wax figurines, their hands can be lifted to any position, and they will hold that position without change for lengthy periods. Prolonged catatonia can lead to muscle breakdown and other complications. Catatonia is therefore considered a psychiatric and a medical emergency.

Cognitive Behavioral Therapy (CBT): This is a very effective therapy that attempts to resolve emotional problems by understanding and removing false or distorted views about self and the world. It exercises to challenge and correct cognitive distortions. CBT can help with problems related to anxiety, depression, and OCD. To some extent, it can even help with some symptoms related to schizophrenia and other psychotic disorders.

Dual Diagnosis and Comorbidity: The coexistence of two or more mental illnesses together such as psychotic disorder and alcohol dependence is said to be dual diagnosis condition. The existence of mental retardation and mental illness is also given the same label of being a dual diagnosis condition. Other combinations can exist. Dual diagnosis tends to be common in institutional settings. Treatment is more complicated in such conditions.

Dual diagnosis and comorbidity exists by some estimates in 40 to 50 percent of those diagnosed with schizophrenia and schizoaffective disorder.

Religion and Other Beliefs shared by a community: Commonly held views in the community and strongly held religious beliefs, even if they appear irrational, are not delusions. They are not grounds for the diagnosis of mental illness.

Depersonalization: A sense of detachment from one's identity. It can be produced in situations of intense stress, under the influence of psychedelic drugs, some prescribed medications or during certain mystical states. It may or may not be a sign of mental illness.

DSM5: This stands for the 5th edition of the *Diagnostic and Statistical Manual* of mental disorders. It is a political, epidemiological and a somewhat scientific document. It is a shared view of what the different categories of mental illness are. The manual is, to some extent, a "committee view" of what the different illness categories should be. It is a guidepost and does serve a useful purpose of standardizing the terms of discussion. It is, however, not to be taken as a bible and is definitely not the end all of our understanding about mental illness. Some sections may even be fictitious.

Echolalia: This is a symptom found in schizophrenia spectrum disorders. It is a condition in which the patient "echoes" or repeats whatever is stated to him or her.

ECT (Electroconvulsive Therapy): This is a form of therapy where a seizure for about one minute is induced by passing weak electrical currents into the brain. The patient is under anesthesia, and the muscles are relaxed. *It is a safe and effective procedure and can be lifesaving.* It is very effective for certain states of catatonia found in schizophrenia. It also provides dramatic benefits for severely depressed patients who have stopped eating are in acute crisis due to their poor nutritional intake. I have seen a malnourished, depressed patient (due to the refusal of food) awaken in a few minutes after ECT and, in recovery, ask where his breakfast is.

The treatment of ECT has been politicized and vilified unjustly due to past misuse in unregulated institutional settings. The procedure is now administered in the operating room of a hospital with the help of anesthesia and muscle relaxation, so that side effects are minimized.

Ego: The rational, logical part of oneself that decides right from wrong. There is more to it, but this is the basic essence. It is derived from what we are told by parents, authority figures and our own rational thinking.

Superego: The imbibed rules and dictates learned in childhood about what constitutes right and wrong. These beliefs are often not fully examined. They dictate our sense of right and wrong. An overly punitive superego may burden the person with a sense of excessive guilt and poor sense of themselves and provide fertile grounds for depression.

Extrapyramidal Symptoms (EPS): This is a group of side effects caused by some antipsychotic medications. These symptoms include one or more of the following: tremors, rigidity of movement and a sense of restlessness. The symptoms are caused by blocking of dopamine receptors in some areas of the brain.

Executive function: The ability to anticipate, plan, and coordinate activities in one's environment for the purpose of achieving certain goals. Executive functioning is the product of the most evolved part of the brain: the frontal lobe.

Any brain disease that affects the frontal lobe can affect executive functioning.

Flashbacks: This is a re-experiencing of a past traumatic event. It can feel very real and as if the event is happening all over again. This symptom is one of the key symptoms in PTSD (Post-Traumatic Stress Disorder).

Flight of ideas: This is a dramatic symptom of the manic state. The patient may talk in rapid fashion about a certain idea and shift directions to start talking about an obliquely related topic and then shift directions again on another tangent. The ideas seem to be in rapid flight and prone to shifting directions. It is different from the loosening of associations because one can still discern the logic of the different thoughts expressed even if they are marginally related to each other.

Id: This is an amalgamated force of our essential drives and passions that motivate us to do all the things we do. This may include our drive for meeting the needs related to sex, food, shelter and security.

Ideas of reference: This is a symptom wherein the person may believe that something pertains to them when it does not. For example, there may be a news article in the paper or a report on TV news that they feel is referring to them specifically. They may also feel that they are receiving special coded messages through the media.

Lability: This is a feature of mania in bipolar disorder. In this the person can quickly change from anger to laughter and friendship or from being friendly to being surly and hostile if their demands and wishes are not met right away. Lability is a term used to describe the ease with which something changes from liquid form to a gas form. Increased lability of affect is a good way to describe the tendency for emotions to change quickly in mania of bipolar disorder.

Loosening of Associations: This is a condition found in severe psychosis such as schizophrenia or schizoaffective disorder. In this, the ideas expressed by the person do not seem to make sense and are not logically connected. When loosening is severe, the words may come out as a stream of unconnected words called a "word salad".

Melancholia: This is on the opposite end of the mood scale to the ecstatic, elevated mood state of mania. In this the patient may experience profound sadness that hangs like a black cloud; their appetite goes down, they may wake up early and may experience symptoms of worthlessness, hopelessness, and nihilism. In severe states, risk for suicide is high and psychotic symptoms with nihilistic themes may emerge. The person may need hospitalization.

ECT is an effective tool for rapid relief of melancholia. The antidepressant medications are also effective, but these take 4 to 6 weeks to show benefit. Sometimes the benefit may start sooner. There may be a higher risk of suicide as the person starts coming out of depression as they may still have suicidal ideations with increased energy and focus to carry out such thoughts and ideations.

Mental Status Exam: This is a snapshot of the person's mental state in the period during the interaction with the clinician. It evaluates the person's appearance, their relatedness, their level of cooperation, and any unusual mannerisms or movements. In addition, it also looks at how they are expressing themselves and if what they generally say makes sense or is difficult to understand. The mental status also examines their affect, which is the range of their emotional expression, their subjective mood state, and any unusual thought content. Their level of orientation, alertness, and speech patterns are also assessed. Any disturbance of thought processes such as loosening or the flight of ideas is also noted in the mental status when found. There are other things such as intelligence that can also be ascertained in the mental status exam of a child or adult.

Mixed states: This is when both depression and mania exist in a patient at the same time.

Mood stabilizer: These are medications that prevent the fluctuations of mood that are seen in bipolar disorder. Some effective mood stabilizers are lithium, divalproic acid (Depakote), and carbamazepine (Tegretol). Some atypical antipsychotic medications such as olanzapine, risperidone, and others have also shown benefit as mood stabilizers. Typical antipsychotics such as haloperidol, fluphenazine, and others are also effective. Antipsychotics were once avoided for bipolar disorder but, if needed, they can be useful.

Negative symptoms: These are symptoms caused by an absence or decrease of normal function. These are found in individuals with schizophrenia. These negative symptoms namely are avolition (lack of drive or initiative), alogia (decreased speech), and a flattening of emotional expression. The negative symptoms also lead to a decrease in activities of daily living such as bathing, brushing teeth, grooming, etc. The person may isolate themselves to a room that becomes progressively disorganized and unkempt.

Neurosis: A condition in which various internal emotional conflicts lead to dysfunctional outward behaviors. Neurosis has the net effect of compromising effectiveness in one's personal and professional life.

Obsessions: These are often irrational and intrusive thoughts that a person seems to have a hard time dislodging from their mind. It is a hallmark of obsessive compulsive disorder. The person may engage in ritualistic behaviors to decrease the intensity of such thoughts, such as repeated handwashing or tapping something a certain number of times. Such ritualistic behaviors are called compulsions and form the other component of obsessive-compulsive disorder.

Paranoia: A state of heightened fear and suspiciousness.

Personality traits: The ways of relating based on certain value sets carried by a person.

Personality Disorder: This is when the habitual way of relating to others or thinking causes conflicts with others. Examples may be the excessive need for personal adoration in narcissism or inflexibility in obsessive-compulsive personality disorder. A borderline personality disorder that switches from idealizing to demonizing those they work with, subsequently acting out in a dramatic manner, is another example. Individuals with antisocial personality disorder lack an inner moral core and tend to exploit others without remorse, repentance or shame. They may violate rules of the law if they think they can get away with it or may not even care about the consequences. They usually fail to learn from their past mistakes.

Perseveration: A tendency to repeat a word or thought. The person has a difficult time switching subjects.

Pharmacogenomics: A field of science that studies the difference in how individuals metabolize drugs and how some individuals are uniquely affected by the different drugs.

Pharmacotherapy: The treatment of psychiatric illness with the help of medications.

Positive symptoms: Symptoms found in schizophrenia and schizoaffective disorder that are not normally present in the normal population. Examples include symptoms such as hallucinations, delusions, and loosening of associations.

Pressured speech: This is a feature of mania when speech output is increased, and words come pouring out like pressured water through a water hose. The person is unable to stop the excessive talking. It is difficult for the listener to get a word in edgewise. If interrupted, the person may get angry due to lability. The speech may also shift directions rapidly due to other manic features such as the flight of ideas and tangentiality.

Psychopath: A psychopath is a person who has no inner sense of right or wrong and does whatever is expedient for his or her interests at the moment. They are remorseless and are immune to all sense of shame. The psychopath has no imbibed sense of right and wrong and may even flaunt society's laws.

Psychosocial stressors: These are events in the social life of the individual that are stressful. This may include happy and sad events such as a marriage, promotion, birth of a child or a loss such as being laid off, divorce or a diagnosis of a terminal illness in a family member.

Psychosis: It is the inability to tell the real from the unreal. For example, the person may feel that aliens have implanted devices in their body, or that a TV news anchor is reading news in a code meant only for them. The person with psychosis can get caught up in delusions and has no insight about the error in their perception. The person cannot be dissuaded by logical entreaties.

Rapid cycling: In bipolar disorder, when mood shifts to either severe depression or mania four or more times in a year, it is called rapid cycling.

Sign: This is something that is evident to observation such as tremor, pacing, loud speech, disorganized speech, the person talking to themselves, or neglect of self-care, etc.

Symptom: This is the problem that the patient describes to you such as not being able to sleep, feeling sad all the time or hearing voices others cannot hear, etc.

Tangentiality: This is a symptom of mania marked by launching of conversations on topics only marginally related to the topic under discussion. The side conversation may be launched by a word or idea that has a very weak and tenuous link with the earlier subject.

Tardive dyskinesia: This is a side effect related to the long term use of antipsychotic medications. The hallmark of this is an abnormal involuntary movement in different parts of the body. Usually, it is first evident in the face or tongue but may involve the limbs or the trunk as well.

Thought blocking: In this the person has difficulty completing his thought and may stop midsentence followed by a long pause. He may resume a different sentence with a different thought or stay quiet. They may not remember what they were talking about. It is a feature of schizophrenia-related thought processes.

CHAPTER 7

EPILOGUE

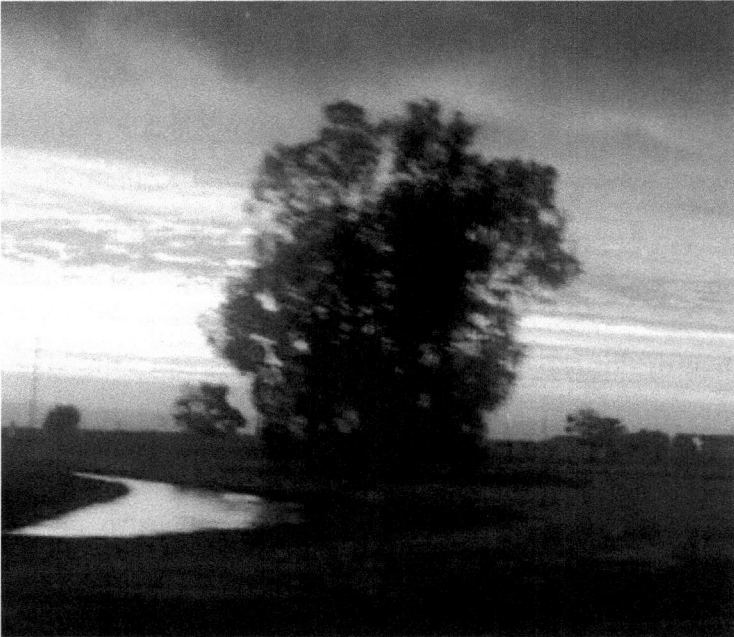

(Near Corcoran, CA)

Final words have a way of not being final. In the discussion on schizophrenia, ultimately, it is the patients and their families that must deal with the illness on a day to day to basis. We have been impressed by their courage and stoicism through the ups and downs. Many can overcome the hurdles posed by a severe illness to reach a place of peace and some tranquility in their lives.

These patients, more than anyone else, have demonstrated that schizophrenia and schizoaffective disorder can be overcome.

Indeed, the outlook for patients with schizophrenia is not as bleak as it was once thought to be. A majority of patients achieve remission of most of their symptoms and can lead fairly productive lives. A third of patients may require a greater level of support, but even they can be stabilized with the right treatment and right environment of care.

In my experience, while a few patients have been intellectually or physically challenged, others have been brilliant or even gifted. One of the patients at a hospital could outwit any member of staff at a game of chess. Other patients had dazzling skills with a simple paper and pen and could effortlessly create exquisite drawings.

The ultimate example of great talent in someone with schizophrenia is represented in the movie "A Beautiful Mind". This movie depicted the life of John Nash. He was a world-class mathematician who saw the unique patterns in everyday life and nature that others did not see.

It shows him grappling with mathematical concepts that later won him the Nobel Prize. It also shows him later getting caught up in a web of conspiracy theories and delusions that drove him further and further from reality until he got on the right medication. Risperidone did wonders for him.

Each patient is unique, with his or her unique life perspective, his or her own dreams, fears, and hopes. Each one is a multifaceted individual.

A person with schizophrenia is not "a schizophrenic" but a person with an illness just as there are other individuals in society with an illness. We do not refer to the person with hypertension as "a hypertensive" but grant them their unique individuality. We should afford the same respect and considerations to those diagnosed with schizophrenia.

These people are just like so many others not diagnosed with schizophrenia. Behind the label are real people who may be full of potential for good.

OTHER BOOKS BY THE AUTHOR

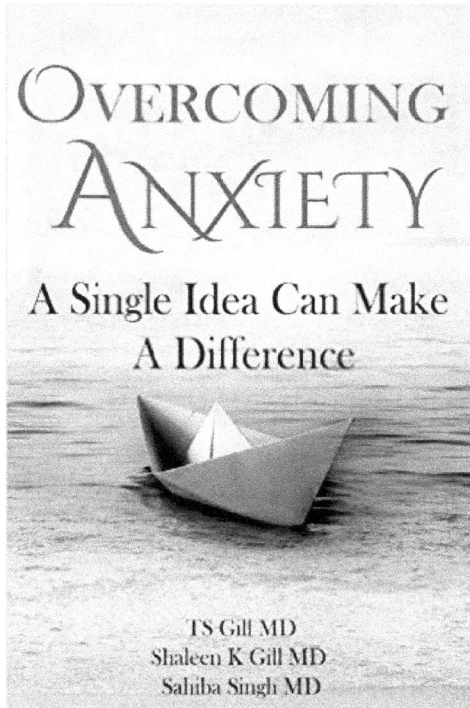

http://www.amazon.com/Overcoming-Anxiety-Single-Idea-Difference/dp/0989664929/ref=sr_1_2?ie=UTF8&qid=14436667 10&sr=8-2&keywords=Tirath+S+Gill+MD

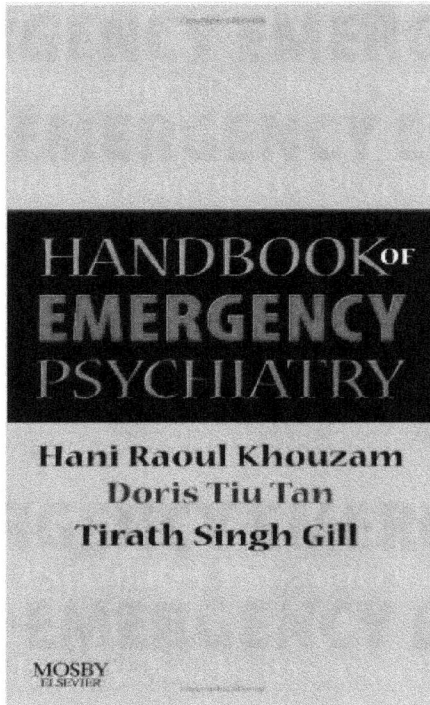

http://www.amazon.com/Handbook-Emergency-Psychiatry-Hani-Khouzam/dp/0323040888/ref=sr_1_4?ie=UTF8&qid=1443666710&sr=8-4&keywords=Tirath+S+Gill+MD

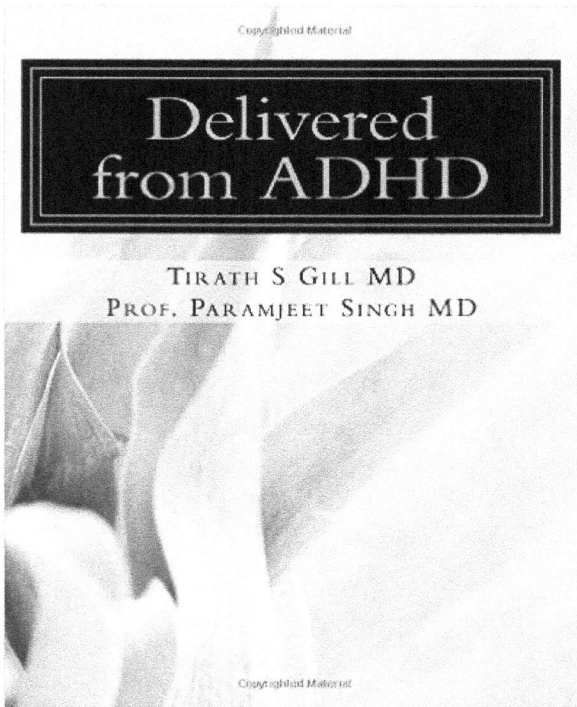

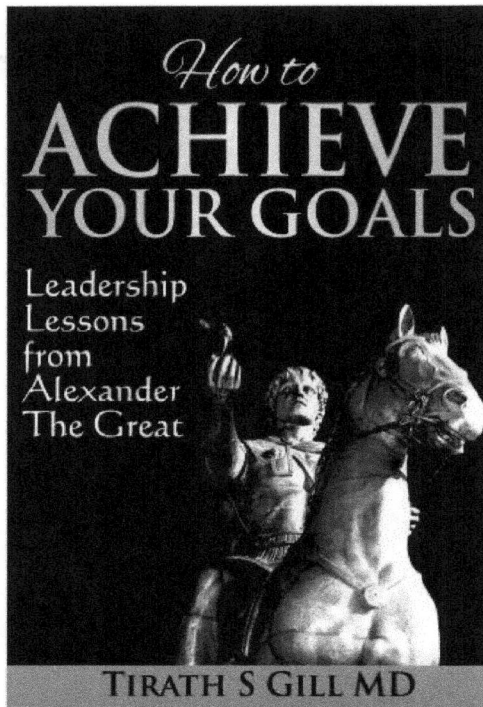

http://www.amazon.com/Achieve-Your-Goals-Tirath-Gill-ebook/dp/B00KTTBCY0/ref=sr_1_fkmr3_3?ie=UTF8&qid=1443666710&sr=8-3-fkmr3&keywords=Tirath+S+Gill+MD

NOTES